Lunacy Lost

Names of individuals have been changed to protect privacy.

"Osage End" represents a composite of experiences
in Emporia, Kansas and Lawrence, Kansas.

ISBN: 1-4681-4654-8
ISBN-13: 9781468146547

Lunacy Lost

Sue Westwind

Dedication

For Starra:
Tell your side someday

Table of Contents

INTRODUCTION

Marie Elton stared at the dust balls revealed by morning light. *How did those get there?* Hugging a baseboard behind the sectional sofa, dirt in corners always accused her. The gray, little puffs marked her secret scorecard: how was she managing the house and family? Marie turned on her heel to find a mop. She was not my mother yet.

Agnes' door was wide open; to Marie, it sounded like the old woman was clearing her throat. Was she congested today? Marie thought she'd check, and padded closer. Now the sound was clipped, random, and distraught. Her mother-in-law was choking to death! The mop handle slapped the hardwood floor as Marie bolted.

Inside the elder's room the bed was in disarray. On top of it Agnes was even more undone. She was not my grandmother yet. But if she'd had her way that morning, we'd have never met.

Agnes Wohler Elton lay across twisted sheets, pillows flung to the corners. Her bathrobe gaped, a nightgown hiking up with the effort she made. Agnes had the robe's terrycloth belt around her throat, pulling it tighter and tighter. She was choking all right, in fits and starts, but seeing Marie and hearing her cry out, having her rush over—it was enough. Agnes stopped yanking and gasping. Marie tore at the belt anyway, freeing it from the soft, creased neck.

Daughter-in-law didn't realize that the deed could not be accomplished. No time to think: how even if a person lost consciousness for a second, the tourniquet on the throat would go slack and breath would rush in. Marie was too innocent to realize you couldn't strangle yourself this way. But Agnes' intention was clear.

Almost a suicide. Here in this house. My house. Marie stood immobilized, unable to help or to hinder the tears of the woman who had birthed the man she loved. It was a twenty-five-year-old day in her life, two years before I was born. For Agnes it was also a first.

Though far from her last cry for help.

❋ ❋ ❋

Most of my life, I've felt captive to the question: what makes mental illness happen? Its specter was ever present at the edges of my family, erupting time and again into catastrophe. My grandmother came to embody this curse, living with us between hospital stays, heiress to those who purposefully ended their own lives. Later, as my older brother grew into a young man, madness stalked him with a powerful stigma: paranoid schizophrenia. When puberty claimed my own body I had a drastic change of mind, and my family saw it as the descent of our genetic disease. I too gained a diagnosis. Then came the children, garnering in short order the labels of their day: autism, attention deficit hyperactivity disorder (ADHD).

Today, I suppose mental health professionals would call me "recovered." I've worked as both a hypnotherapist and as a Holistic Mental Health Coach, grateful for students and clients who've taught me volumes. I question Big Pharma's proclamation that medication is the answer, for reasons made loud and clear in this book. Yet despite the great failure of antidepressants and antipsychotics, despite the immoral antics of the pharmaceutical industry, its dominion goes largely uncontested. Sadly, the record of over 400 modes of psychotherapy is also spotty.

No one chooses the conditions into which one is born. Though it may be inauspicious to sound a note of confinement at the outset, the absence of freedom (and justice) for sufferers of emotional and behavioral disorders is a theme that won't go away. Whether the jail is literal, electrical (as in shock treatments), surgical, or pharmaceutical, the emancipation that a cure would bring is not on psychiatry's wish list.

Yet there is a model for real change. Within the autism community, I found a steady and growing, parent-led march to find answers and reverse the diagnosis. I found a partnership between practitioners and family members that is unequaled. My daughter finally began to make strides to health, and I put the new information to work for me.

What I ultimately discovered is that a full turnaround from abject mental pain is possible—not just for a few, but for many. I would never have been lucky enough to become well if not for the efforts of the cutting-edge world of autism advocacy. At first, I thought it was all for Nina. But the foment of honest seeking for the root causes of autism turned out to be a gift to her parent as well.

In my case, healing was exhilarating and profound. I had not logged years of psychiatric drug use. Decades of pain, hiding, addiction, codependency, labels and more labels, countless therapy sessions, and chronic physical limitations? That pretty much sums up my struggle.

Within a relatively short time of whirlwind study and experimentation, it became clear what had been messing with me. I finally reached an experience of health that, as the saying goes, hit on all cylinders. I had already learned much from autism parents who were savvy about everything from homeopathy to hyperbarics. Thanks to the Internet, I excitedly connected with people around the globe who had discovered that nature's tools—even in cases where soul-numbing prescriptions had ruled a person for years—could release the body and mind into a freedom where justice comes from just saying "no" to Pharma's drugs.

The concept that the body's travails strongly affect the mind is given lip service, but never invited to take part in a badly needed overhaul of the mental health system. We can learn from the autism world, where parents took the bull by the horns and the professionals followed. Not that there is any lack of research or success stories regarding alternative medicine for depression, anxiety, schizophrenia, and bipolar disorder. For those who wish to go the natural route, many books and websites have been made available by knowledgeable holistic practitioners who want with all their hearts to help. They are my inspiration. But I'm here to share a story, not a step-by-step treatment plan.

Dr. Lewis Mehl-Madrona, of Lakota and Cherokee heritage and author of *Coyote Medicine*, pleads for a medicine based on narrative. He says we need stories that work. In indigenous cultures, stories are the mainstay of healing, transferring the balm made of insight and hope. So I turned to the vehicle of memoir that asks: have you been there too? Would you like to envision a better way? **Lunacy Lost** tells of my quest to fathom the true nature of the beastly epidemic we call "mental illness." Its genuine roots—and a blueprint for healing—were revealed to me by a child so baffling that at first I wondered if I could parent her. What a mistake that would have been: missing out on the largest lesson of my life.

Is there anyone, deep down, who doesn't wonder where such widespread health problems will take humanity? We are depressed, stressed, ADDed, and OCDed, addicted to bad food, synthetic chemicals, and computer screens. Can a new drug or reworked form of therapy possibly save us? I propose that instead we set aside the glorification of the disembodied mind. We need a sweeping reset of our assumptions about the body, the spirit, and the planet's role in the arena of emotion, thought, and behavior—all those intangibles that we've been taught to keep private, separate, to shoulder as our unique cross to bear. I call this approach The Nutrient Path (others use the phrase Green Mental Health) and it's rising and spreading, doing countless minds good. However, "one size fits all" does not apply.

In my opinion, our mental health crisis only *seems* unfathomable. The problem lies with a weave of long-standing assumptions from without and within.

First of all, there is the professional milieu that manipulates our views, making a specialty of mind without telling us precisely what *is* mind or mental health. The professionals' tools for the brain are the endlessly diversified antidepressants and antipsychotics, courtesy of Big Pharma. The side effects of these products often replace or undermine the work of soulful talk that therapy should offer in our healing process. Unfortunately, many therapists tout mere cognitive re-structuring as the fix for a body-mind on the fritz.

Secondly, there are religious traditions that separate the shining key—knowledge of the *whole* body—from any discussion of mental healing, peddling dogmas that label our bodies (from the neck down) as the site of sin. Although post-modern threads of reform are welcome news, all of the major religions historically promote this divisiveness by exhorting us to save the spirit while downplaying, if not outright despising, the flesh.

Thirdly, there is the weight of our worst stories—real traumas suffered in the span of many relationships. The closing decades of the last century exploded with revelations about how families fall apart: gender wars, predators and perpetrators, patterns of abuse passed down the generations. With such horrors close at hand, many can't get past the art of blaming to see that forgiveness is more than an act of will. Forgiveness and moving on come naturally when we take a planetary view of what most likely is causing "mental" illness to spread across humanity.

Prozac deficiencies in unbalanced brains, sinners who should transcend the flesh, or heaps of familial hurt—these are the stories that have not worked. What else might contribute to the swelling ranks of the anxious, the bipolar, and the schizoaffective, to the many children who can't learn, can't talk, and don't even know why they feel what they feel?

✻ ✻ ✻

Out of love, I went looking early for answers to this question. For thirteen years, my sweet-faced, songstress grandmother lived with our family. She was, by all accepted definitions, crazy. From time to time she endured 1950's-style locked wards and electroshock treatments, dutifully took her meds, and then came back to me, the only person in our household who loved her without ambivalence. This book begins with her, because she was the one who dragged our family lineage of failed brains and unspoken heartache right into the living room.

As a teenager I came to believe that my grandmother's agony was the result of what she saw: three beloved family members who died on her. Long after she left us, I grieved helplessly for her losses. Then, as a young woman buoyed by the countercultural wave and the rhetoric of women's liberation, I grasped that the poor thing was powerless, a girl and then a wife without options, and I raged at patriarchy on her behalf.

But follow in her footsteps I did. During one of many breakdowns I turned to the spirit, thinking that the divine might save me from the ranks of family members who had faltered—all church-going agnostics, disdainful of mystic abandon. I thought I had found the answer when I experienced a spiritual awakening to the Divine Feminine that righted my life's zigzag course in so many ways. Yet the transformation was incomplete. When my first child was diagnosed with a fate more cruel than our family disease, I turned away from the Source whom I imagined had dealt this blow. Throughout the bulk of this narrative, my "crisis of faith" plays its minor key, resolving itself at last through a most unexpected development. I like to think my "crazy" ancestors would approve of the peace I finally made with a Deeper Power, rooted in earth and sky.

Still, I kept asking where our family disease came from. What accounted for subsequent generations' withdrawal from life, their pernicious restraint, a billowing silence and depression, an escape to fatigue and fantasy and the fear of what lay beyond familiar four walls? Were those of us who succumbed simply born weak, sensitive, defective?

Counter to the story of our brokenness is the tale of our famous ancestor, a research scientist who in the 1800's made an accidental discovery that toppled the way his world looked at living and non-living organisms. How could he be so brilliant and productive, while we are so afflicted? What happened to us? Just exactly when did the Wohler Madness begin?

I never considered whether something more concrete might lie behind our troubles. My family believes that our nutcases are simply not wired correctly—the bad brain. But could there be roots that reach *beyond the brain?* There was, and still is, a disinclination to believe that powerful, everyday forces within our bodies—endocrine, digestive, or immune systems—could spark the tongue of eloquent madness. Hold on, we say, that's the domain of other specialists.

I kept uneasy company with the notion that our family disease was "genetic": an inborn, invisible weakness of neural conduits making for emotional strain and muddled thought, a bad luck of the draw. Everyone in the family accepted this as our inconsistent fate, and each wished fervently to be spared. For too long my personal quest was to dodge the bullet any way I could.

It wasn't until I experienced my own daughter's tragedy and her road to healing that I dared to entertain *this* renegade thought about the family disease: what if something man-made and dangerous, not some defect of character, got into our DNA, *and maybe it needn't have been so?* I learned about epigenetics: how environmental insults like toxins can change genetics quickly from one generation to the next. I learned that what we inherit isn't a personal, indelible blueprint, but that *toxins actually interfere with the way genes are expressed.* The whacked genes lose their ability to detoxify a body and its neural net under attack. The result is any number of physiological and mental chronic disorders.

This was the science I never saw coming.

Sparked to go beyond illness of mind and beyond my peculiar clan, I awoke to the fact that my family is not alone in facing basic health questions daily. How do we cope? Will we ever be well? Today, we might say that many a family story of mental illness is not merely about the brain, bad luck, or bad behavior. It is about what our world is becoming.

I dare to speculate thus because of a gorgeous, quirky, loving infant adopted by my husband and I, and diagnosed with autism in her second year of life. Sure, I was primed not to give up on my kid: after what happened to me, I never trusted psychiatry's "biochemical imbalance" theory. But I know what I saw when nutrients, diet changes, and detox were deployed against a disorder considered hopeless and incurable. My experience in parenting such a child is far from singular. I owe deep gratitude to the mother-warriors, to the researchers with the guts to keep after the truth, and to the dedicated clinicians who refused to believe that autistic persons were simply another flavor of crazy. They went through the body to reach the mind, and there struck the gold of knowledge for all to share.

The pieces fit: my bloodline's inability to relate effectively, our toxic world at large, and the rising number of children saddled with violent behavior and learning disabilities. The latter grow into distracted, depressed, and antisocial adults. What this correlation taught me was that my family disease turned out to be more than a dreaded inheritance of a failure to buck up and be productive. The proof I had every day before me was the similarities between my afflictions and those of my *adopted* child. No genetic material shared—yet we both fought our way out of scary places together, using the same nourishments as tools.

Nina (as I call her here), a child with autism, led me to this treasure trove of truth. This is not another story about a recovered kid, though miracles abound in these pages. This is about my recovery, and how Nina made it happen for me.

I've spent decades either stalking the cause or trying to outrun my family curse, which meant that for a long time I ran from family, from psychiatry, and from the status quo. Come meet the members of my afflicted clan and bear with me until I finally understand them. Take a look at the early days of anti-psychiatry, when "the mentally ill" exalted madness as a political act; witness the hunt for the crazy-makers among suspects galore. Join me during the first flush of the New Age, when permission was granted to explore consciousness without drugs, prescribed or not, and see how sensitive minds widened—until, in my case, the body demanded its say.

Then meet Nina, who saved my life.

Our children, the fastest growing "consumers" of mental health services and medication, are the signposts of a dangerous future. I know because, you see, there was this baby. She was beautiful, and she was mine. Then she became very sick, very silent, and very sad. Our double healing—like those of many mothers and children who forbear on the nutrient path—contains the seeds to do away with "mental illness" and "behavior disorders" forever.

We *can* give up madness.

PART ONE
LUNACY'S LINEAGE

Chapter 1
THE WOHLER MADNESS

Thwack. Thwack. SMACK.

Rhythm made the sound, but anger pushed it too. The house never held a beat like that. Pulled by the wants of a five-year-old— sugar and starch shaped into snacks, plus finding my friends on a side- walk past home—that *SMACK, swish, CRACK!* called louder. Something was going on in the bottom of the house.

I seldom played in that belowground expanse with the pimply walls, dim and damp. Ours was a basement, but farm relatives called theirs a cellar. The only word that formed as I searched out those rhyth- mic wallops was: *Who?*

I paused in the kitchen, the room of women. Its color was meant to lift you up. Being five in 1959, I took for granted the cheery-bright themes in tract homes at this edge of a nearly southern city. Sunny kitchens spread light from a wide window over the sink where moth- ers toiled in suds, always home, for where else would they be? Outside, grills and chaise lounges were measured against the ones next door, and wasn't the size of the patio up for comparison too? My mother could have cared less about any of it as she made her moves in the basement, square jaw clenching back every word.

I sat down in that kitchen, emptied of adults for the moment, still feeling torn between the thunking plunks coming from below and the desire to head outside with a handful of pretzels. Out where the apron strings loosened for a spell, because "out" was the sitter that every mom counted on. Nature was my yard, where the next yard and friends' back yards merged into one block, indivisible, with sameness and covert competition for all. Nature was also the vacant lot, a "For Sale" sign stuck in its side, waiting for new lumber and glass. When the skeleton frame was up and silent, in the evenings after the crew left, so what if a few kids stomped and yelled through walls-to-be? Nature sat still, a yard-to-be.

I knew a place like that, and I knew who would be there now, watchful on the edges, waiting for quittin' time, clutching their Bit O' Honeys or wearing Fritos like diamond rings on spindly fingers. But there was that sound, right below my feet. Where *was* my mom, anyway?

Marie Elton endured.

As cook, cleaner, and head of nothing she deemed important, she aspired to be well liked by the smart people she feared surpassed her. Publicly, she agreed that marriage and motherhood were her crowning achievement. She called it her career. Too bad the heaveho of every day was so, well, boring. It pained her that her sacrifice to overcome clutter and grime went unnoticed. She longed for the white-picket-fence version of family life as seen in her women's magazines, complete with appreciative children and a predictable spouse. Like her peers in their yellow kitchens, she worked hard to embrace parenting as a full-time vocation, quick to say she was a big giant nobody until she became a *mom*, the 1950's female fulfillment. Except for one thing. And that one thing threatened to ruin her day, again.

Because of the woman who lived upstairs in her otherwise acceptable middle-class house, my mother knew that her life would never match the going pictures of bliss. She and my dad uneasily accepted the fact that they harbored a madwoman. To me she was Grandma, and the best one at that. When we weren't outside with nature for a babysitter, my brother and I had the madwoman. *Blood is thicker than water*, my mother used to sigh, and then shake her head. I used to wonder why this meant that my grandmother had to live with us, because real blood was not so thick—it spurted and ran, scary bright red, and water had nothing to do with it.

But a live-in mother-in-law was not in Marie Elton's script. Every day my thoroughly Catholic mom brushed her auburn hair while leaning over a tiny crucifix attached to the rosary she never said. No time to pray. Her man would have smiled at prayers in the house anyway—and not the pleased smile, but the other one. The rosary lay on her dresser, and maybe she thought doing her hair over the beads mattered to God. Because at dawn, before any inhabitant on two floors had yet stirred, she really thought she could handle the madwoman snoring at the top of the stairs.

Not that housing my Gram was part of the original matrimonial deal. But in *sweet innocent Marie* the other relatives saw an opportunity to foist their responsibilities elsewhere. So my Grandma Elton came to live with us, because there was no other place for her to go.

Except when she was really, for all intents and purposes, already gone.

Mentally ill, whispered the adults. *Not all here.* I didn't know what they meant, and I didn't care. But when the whispers started, it meant my mom would get a break, a vacation in which to believe the white-picket-fence perfection was hers for a short time, removed from an old woman's misfortune and malaise.

Listening to the blows coming from somewhere beneath my feet, I recalled seeing my mother earlier that day with a grim face. She tackled the domestic routine with a small scarf knotted in front, à la Lucille Ball, and red lipstick that blared from dawn rising to cold-cream night. When she went down into the coolness of that great below, she left the door gaping wide open. The *thwack*—pause—*thwack-smack-you-awful-thing* sent an ominous message to my little-girl senses as I peered into the darkness below.

My mom always turned on the lights to do laundry, but I couldn't hear the humming drums turning any trousers. The bare bulbs dotting the space were cold. Grimy windows at either end were little help, but the yellow kitchen beamed down all the light she needed.

Then I saw her, after my first downward step, because her targets were dead ahead. They seemed so innocent—what could they have done to her? There, at the foot of the stairs, was my mother, hurling books with all her might and, before I got there, without a trace of shame.

Her victims were books. And that wasn't right.

Scattered on the floor were the *Harvard Classics* from my father's study, now no longer considered worthy of daylight. Compact and scarlet, lettered in gold, they came off the shelves as if their bearer could not help it, as if she could divest all those choked up, can't-do-anything-about-it, here-we-go-again feelings into a pile of haughty books brought low. A thud here, splayed pages there: it seemed to satisfy her, to erase for a moment the central fact of her suburban life—that lunatic on the top floor was driving her crazy.

"What are you—?"

Mur looked up, defiant, trapped. That's what we called her: *Mur.* As a barely talking toddler, I couldn't say *Mother.* "Mur" made my father laugh and the short syllable stuck.

But in the basement, throwing books, Mur didn't look like herself. Not like when she picked up the toys in our rooms, making order two steps behind our thoughtlessness. Now she was deliberately making a mess! Was it a joke?

"She makes me so angry!" spat Marie, aka Mur, with her trademark mix of nerve wrestling with guilt—a mix that was contagious and far too simple to learn. Was it the title of the books that made her pick them? *Harvard Classics.* I'd heard that word *Harvard* before.

At one time *Harvard* was a powerful mantra in our tract home in Kentucky, a word infused with hope that we would move "up." Up to Boston, to become one with this Harvard University, but until then my father said, *don't tell anyone!* My parents worked and reworked the words throughout the house: Boston, Harvard, Boston, Harvard. It was my first introduction to the texture of dread.

My father ached to leave our nearly southern city. There were the irritating, slow drawls of his colleagues, the discomfort of segregation, and his own ho-hum prospects for academic advancement. My mother hoped for greater adventure and a bigger house. My *I'd rather die!* response was about losing the only friends and school culture I'd ever known. After I'd blabbed to the entire neighborhood anyway, the name of the city and the university were never said again. We were staying, it seemed, for now. There would be no Harvard, and I wondered if it was because I had—far and wide—told.

They'd almost made it. My parents believed that the madwoman whose moods they monitored daily would disappear once they joined the intellectual elite of New England. I would lose my southern accent as soon as we lost my grandmother. Not that Louisville was bad. It was a city, after all, nothing like the Oklahoma farm my mother gladly escaped, and a far cry from the tiny Kansas town where the madwoman upstairs, Agnes Wohler Elton, inherited the family disease.

"Your grandma is such a *martyr*," my mother said at last. She bent to stack the books back on the shelf in the proper way, shame searing her eyes. This always meant that I would hurt because she did, because I played some part in her despair. "I'm a bad mother," she would often cry, hiding in the bathroom with tears ravaging mascara into big shiners on her cheeks.

"You're not! You're not!" I'd protest, falling into some hole I knew should not be there. Now I'd caught her in her secret basement explosion, and she grasped what a lasting impression this would make on me. The hole that was my helplessness got bigger, while the basement contained a display of emotion we both knew should not see the light of day.

I watched my mother stuff errant curls back into her scarf. Thanks to the yellow kitchen light, I beheld an unusual sight: there were no tears this time. She'd had a temper tantrum, and I learned how adults do it. They could blow their lids about other adults! This was new information, an education for an almost-first-grader full of her importance now that she was about to climb aboard the long yellow bus headed for school.

There was only one thing I needed to know, even if it steamed her all over again. My parents were always free with new words, and they seemed to like it when we pressed them for the meanings. Words (as I gathered from her book-throwing), especially those said with a certain tone, were so special that they probably came from pages of print bound by spines with bold lettering. My dad taught his students some ways with words: how to wrangle them into the kind of magic that just might, one day, make a *Harvard Classic*. Now the word of the day had attached itself to someone I regarded with an admiration so uncomplicated that I itched to get the scoop on it.

"What's a martyr?

The madwoman above

Upstairs, Agnes Elton (maiden name Wohler) kept her quarters pin-neat and sunlit as any pastel kitchen. The extra light came in handy for illuminating sheet music of all types. Marked by her many absences from our home, she was also set apart by her music.

With a gift none of us could fathom, Agnes brought forth huge chords, meaty with reverb, from an old upright piano that dominated her room. It was something my grandmother shared with me alone on bright mornings when my brother was off with his lunchbox to school. Mur hung laundry or vacuumed in her pedal pushers—lonely and yet, given the options, glad to be alone. My father, Agnes' son, would reappear before supper with the energy of the outside world in tow. But not once did the whole family ever climb the stairs for a concert. The madwoman's music was all mine.

Agnes might have been the in-law, the burden, the nut in the attic, but for me she buffered the shock waves of family life and received my constant company for thanks. Sitting on the piano bench at her side or pinching the chenille on her bedspread, I studied the alchemy of rouge and powder on cheeks that were soft and kissable. She played dreamy and slow, and sang a smooth soprano. Agnes and her sister, Antonia, a violinist, used to work at parties and receptions in their youth to earn a bit of money and some local fame. In those sweet days, the Elton man who would come courting Antonia and fill their worlds was still unknown. Even more unimaginable, then, was that Antonia would up and die on her, and that life would come down to this: shuttled among her grown children for as long as each one could take it.

Given her martyrdom and all.

After showcasing the songs she loved, trilling the likes of "Sentimental Journey" at the keys, the record player came out and glossy 45's went round the turntable. "You ain't nothin' but a hound dog," she'd belt out with Elvis. She charged from genre to genre with a smile that said *any tune's game!* I begged for more, never realizing that big things ailed my best buddy, or that it had all started long ago.

I depended on Grandma Agnes whenever my parents broadcasted how vexed to maximum capacity they were, warning us they were about to blow. Then it would be time for the three of us—my brother Sam, Agnes, and me—to go out. Past the neighborhood, into the foreign swirl. That is, if Agnes was well. If Agnes was home.

We'd take a bus deep into the city to watch first-run movies like *The King and I*. Agnes' powdered face was smooth in the flickering light. She knew all the lyrics and hummed softly as we tracked the story, accomplices to too much fun. Then on to the Blue Boar Cafeteria, where we chose from an array of plated novelties displayed under lamps or arranged on ice. By the time she steered us back onto the bus, we were fat and happy. My parents trusted her with us. Was that crazy, or just an oversight? Or was it recognition that she was really two persons in one—and they knew who would show up when?

❋ ❋ ❋

It's a habit of mine, raking through these memories of the lovable grandma for something that might stand out as real madness. Where was it? How did I miss it? My parents lived with it, shielded it from us, and finally removed it when the time came. Meanwhile, the family disease simmered at the edge of every word spoken, every action taken by my grandmother, whom they seemed to feel was their incarnate cross to bear.

Much later, I put it all together. Agnes Wohler counted herself among the failures of our clan, those so sad that they became mad and prayed not to become the ones who died by their own hand. At least the suicides were few, though persistent in the bloodline. Others in the family did all right, like the famous ancestor who turned out to be more than all right—our star. He was Agnes' uncle...or was it grandfather? My dad could not decide. He had bigger things to dwell on, like how to ascend to a greatness that was, if not untouchable, at least bearable and worthy of defense.

We often visited my mother's relatives, and occasionally my dad's brothers, but I rarely saw an elder who had lived through the Wohler problem. Where were the Wohlers? No holidays, no trans-generational reunions, not a word. How many of them had outrun the family disease? How many were caught? Later I wondered why, as descendants of a scientist who had made such a noteworthy discovery, they weren't proud to congregate. Maybe embarrassment over their sad ones, their mad ones, cancelled out family pride. But the famous Wohler left his mark. If he could stumble his way into recognition as a brain that excels, so could any of us.

Later still, I would ponder why Agnes Wohler didn't use her super-smart relative's glory to hoist her own sense of worth. But she wasn't one to bask in anyone's reflection, not even that of the husband who died on her. One might say that she was too immersed in her own poisonous self-image to allow osmosis with the good. (Wait a minute—women born in 1905 were not allowed a "self-image.") I ended up supposing that my grandmother, quick to turn a scathing eye upon herself, assumed a position so far beneath her famous ancestor that she never spoke of him, out of either reverence or fear.

For our young family, Friedrich Wohler was merely incidental. Some old scientist who lived eons ago in Germany didn't fit our fifties lifestyle, although my brother Sam would increasingly become obsessed with his work. Maybe, because the gent wasn't literary, he left my English Department father unimpressed. Maybe it was because Friedrich Wohler had started out as a medical doctor (once upon a time every male Elton was instructed to become a doctor), but my father had not toed that line. Maybe, because Friedrich was connected to Agnes, there was danger implied: the danger known as the Wohler Madness.

On the other hand, the scientist's deeds could have fueled my father's fire, prompting him to remind us, to repeat the litany: *we are smarter than the average bear, smarter than the average bear.* Because when you were smart you had a fighting chance, the makings of a winner. Our losers had no kick-start to their brains. Their slogan rang out all too clear: *Woe is me, me, me.*

My mother spent a lot of time wishing that her mother-in-law could keep herself in check. Instead, tears leaked from the seams of Agnes' rootless soul. This was too at odds with the social contract: you *had to* buck up, and if you could not do it you made people uncomfortable. Besides, when all was prosperity and progress, whatever was there to be sad about?

My parents were bent on conveying the appearance of happiness. Their emotional leakage was of a different stripe: the righteous anger and bitchery of the breadwinning unit.

And they took seriously their entitlement to vent. Getting goddamn mad was nothing like going insanely mad. How delightfully my parents were set free with permission from company—with or without drinks. I loved to listen, out of sight, and hear my father laugh, hear him tease and cajole, his warmth toward people wafting from his bourbon into the shared air. When the group turned to kvetching it was loud but laced with camaraderie. Everybody joined in.

But that wasn't often. Around his kids, Robert Elton was usually distracted and withdrawn into his own mind. He had work to do. With his wife, he was ever prone to fanning the fires. With Agnes he was hushed, as if ashamed. He knew all her siblings had it, *the mental trouble*. No one had ever cured the Wohler Madness.

❋ ❋ ❋

Whenever anything went wrong, somehow Agnes was to blame.

Like when the coffeepot fell on my mother's toe, fell hard, left an ugly brown splash against the yellow walls. My father offered to help and picked up the pieces. But the looks and the bickering that accompanied it were classic Elton rage-and-blame. The volume was turned low, however. Agnes was upstairs.

There were words uttered about who'd placed the contraption where, how it never sat right anyway, how the cord took over the counter top, eating up valuable space. No one came right to the point, but all the drama was in the faces. Mur's face said:

Now see what happened, see what went out of control when control is all we hope to have, see what you made me do because you ask too much of me and I am resentful, resentful of the endless coffee, the cleaning of the pot, and the hundred other stupid tasks—and now the inconvenience, the damn thing, scalding and bruising my red-lacquered nail… and my crazy mother-in-law living here on top of it too!

But Robert was madder, upper hand mad, as he tried to resurrect the vessel while leaving the cleaning up to her. *Don't bother me with small potatoes, can't you see how much I have to do, someone upstairs is probably listening, clucking her tongue, don't we have enough pain and suffering here?*

For days my mother limped around the kitchen, throwing baleful looks at the percolator. The brew was dutifully poured, but somehow never made it to the table until my father threw down his newspaper and rose dramatically to fetch it himself.

And I learned, once again, how the real world got things done. You had to scream against madness to prove you were immune. Such was not the way of gentle Agnes—but she, they said, was so `clearly helpless, so run out of fuel, her few weak sparks spent on whiny manipulation.

"She's so passive-aggressive!" I overheard my mother say one evening while I drew pictures and Sam pored over his long division. Mur had been reading an abridged account of Freud's theories applied to modern families by *Reader's Digest*. My father was silent, out of his league. Freud wasn't Falkner. Freud made him squirm.

"You ask her *not* to do something, and it's all in the tone of voice: *'Oh'…head bowed…'okay…well I was just trying to…'* Fill in the blank! And then the sorry sniffles! I asked her not to pick up the kids' toys—I said I'd do it. I asked her to please let me decide where the linens go in the closet. If I want to reorganize shelves, I'll do it during spring cleaning. I wish she would just butt out of my affairs! She had her chance to run a home and family, why can't she let me run mine?"

My father simply looked up over his glasses. *That was a long speech*, his piercing blue eyes said.

Decades later, I asked my mother why our boarder's desire to help was crazy. This warranted a mental hospital? "What got your goat most about Grandma? What was it between you two? I mean, besides having to deal with her when she went bonkers." After a few variations on the martyr theme, my mother's proud summary unfurled: "I wouldn't let her do anything!"

"What do you mean, 'anything'?"

"I mean around the house, you know. She did watch you kids, but I chalked that up to grandparent visit-time. She wanted to cook meals, wash loads of clothes, dust the furniture every day. I wasn't having it!"

I stared back in disbelief. "Let me get this straight. Here was a widow who only wanted to fit into her extended family, to be of use, to help *you*—and what did you want her to do, sit in her room all day and be quiet?"

My mother let her shoulders go, in that beat-but-wait-a-minute style. "It wasn't so simple. Why do you think she got thrown out of everybody else's houses? She'd toil away at their chores and then complain it was killing her. If she picked up a piece of lint, she had to tell you about it. Why do you think Aunt Marge sent her away? Grandma told everyone Aunt Marge was working her too hard."

"*I need to be needed.*" My mother spat out Agnes' refrain in disgust.

By now I had taken on the role of advocate—anything to trounce my Mur. "Couldn't you have let her feel needed somehow?"

But the terrycloth-chokehold wasn't the only day of strange that Marie Elton endured.

"The next thing you know, she'd be running outside in her nightgown. I had to chase her around the house like that a time or two. I guess the neighbors were glad we moved."

To litter the street

When the sweet or sassy music upstairs began to fade, my parents' apprehension grew . Next came weeks of creeping, ever-darkening depression: Agnes would sit with her shoulders like shutters trying to close over her chest. The sighs were frequent and long, the line between martyrdom and madness flexing. Why didn't I notice? Was I too young to detect the magnitude of her blues? Or did she rally to my childish regard, faking us both out until I ran off and played somewhere else?

Meanwhile, the show of family life went on as best it could. My brother and I flew below radar, one day tumbling into the next. For my parents, dread gathered itself into well-laid plans for the hour when things would come to a head.

In the midday suburbs of a nearly southern city, Robert and Marie Elton only wanted a life like everybody else on the block. Then along came real madness, a legendary wrench in the works. To make things worse, it came speaking in tongues.

The language Agnes used as she broke apart was English, all right, but it was the King James Version. Her penchant was for stern, Old Testament quotations centered on the unfaithfulness of husband and wives. *Adultery*, Agnes reminded the adults, *was the sin of all sins.* This was embarrassing talk at the breakfast table.

We didn't read Bibles in our house; we preferred to do catechism in other buildings. Sam and I went to Catholic school, and each Sunday the four of us took in the mass as required. But the heavy, leather-bound, fine print, too-cryptic Bible? When Agnes started to slip, her text of choice puzzled my parents. They preferred to sit beneath their brass lamps reading the latest Book-of-the-Month-Club selection or *Life* magazine. The only talk of adultery was on "Perry Mason" after dark.

But they did know that a louder cry for help would come, the last straw. No one wanted to see the woman trying to strangle herself, ever again. That was so far afield from Marie Elton's white-picket dream that she'd buried the memory. But with all the Bible quotes about holy infidelity, madness threatened to erupt like smoke and ashes. What started out as a nice Saturday was about to turn grim. She shook her head. The Wohler Madness was genetic, and could not be cured.

It was my father's duty to speak to his mother about kindly taking her mind and its trappings elsewhere, after first checking to see that the kids were outdoors. With a look, he indicated to his spouse: *it's time.*

Mur would pack up Agnes' bags. Two worlds met over those suitcases, the Lutherans and the Catholics tallying the other's faults. Agnes made it to church irregularly, despite her taste for scriptural gloom and doom. My mother imbibed the mass as a born Irish Catholic, and Robert Elton had converted upon their marriage. He accompanied us on Sundays with an air of silent daydreaming. My brother and I were assured that he took Holy Communion the requisite once a year and confessed his sins as needed. We never saw it.

Later, I learned that being Protestant was as distasteful as going insane. We were drilled in first grade about who made it into heaven.

Apparently the sign on the pearly gates read "For Catholics Only." Agnes, I realized in dismay, was bound for hell.

My mother knew right where to look for the luggage. Agnes, at this point, was pulling it out every other day and morosely announcing her departure—"since I'm so much trouble to everyone," she wept. Her daughter-in-law, five-foot two-inches tall, with a bubble of naturally red hair (and not-a-Wohler, not well versed in abnormal psychology) maneuvered the suitcases onto Agnes' bed while my father coaxed the sad woman downstairs.

"Nothing like this would ever happen down home," Mur muttered. Her solid old aunts and uncles, all unmarried, lived together in the house where they grew up. Her parents still farmed each day and often into the night. There, stiff upper lips said only prayers.

Down home was what they called the Oklahoma homestead that her family tamed and made into the Finley farm. On my father's side, there was nothing like it. Down home meant everything that predated Robert Elton, who came with his mad mother as part of the deal.

Mur hoisted the suitcases onto the bed and glanced ruefully at the gleaming piano keys. She envied talent, in contrast to what she perceived as her ordinary, not awfully smart, self. Yet what good was it, the Wohler smarts? You tinkle the ivories like angels dancing and then end up behind iron bars? Marie winced every time she saw the somber grates covering the state hospital windows. Jail, that's what it was, or worse—at least uppity criminals would fight, spit, and kick for their self-preservation. My mother knew what would happen at the hospital. Agnes would simply give up and they would do to her whatever they did there. It would be torture to visit her until she started talking sense again.

Packing stockings and slips, and thinking of Agnes at home and away, Mur knew that a mother-in-law was forever. So she tucked the Bible under a nightgown and hoped. Hoped that Agnes would find the right line in the Book, and cut the melodrama. Surely, somewhere in those respectable, unreadable pages, the old woman would find peace—and then learn how to live in a nice apartment of her own.

"Adultery is the greatest sin. Jezebel paid," announced Agnes Wohler Elton, her voice shaking as her bags came down the stairs. The biblical Jezebel—Agnes was stuck on her name and her fate. But my grandma, no Jezebel, could not help whom she loved, her favorite sister's beau. Such was the ailing root, the lovesick heart of the matter: Agnes got her dead sister's man. Antonia died in childbirth, leaving the boy for Agnes to raise and the father for her to marry.

Did she think herself a Jezebel because she coveted what was not hers from the very moment the worldly Elton man walked into their house? Was theirs an immediate attraction, or did it slowly gain strength because it was closeted from Antonia's awareness—a fruit so forbidden it thrived on the energy it took to suppress the vine? Or did Agnes and brother-in-law have an understanding that someday they would unite, and was that understanding nurtured even during the marriage and pregnancy that was Antonia's glory?

Or did something happen that only Agnes was left to secret inside? Was there a sin so mortal that Lutherans and Catholics alike would condemn it?

The death of her sister brought Agnes Wohler visions of the wedding altar. Or was she already feeling entitled? After decorum dictated a pause, Agnes told her dead sister's husband, "I do." Whereupon, a few years later, he died too.

So this was her punishment. Jezebel! The man was ever Antonia's. The childbed death worked a bad thought into Agnes' head: she had killed her own sister with a secret desire.

She never told her sons why she always consented to go to the madhouse. Maybe it was her penance, another load due, especially when it came in the form of jolts that shook teeth, skeleton, and bowels—shock treatments as frequent as scheduling allowed. Agnes reveled in her loss of memory afterwards. All trace of Bible quotes was gone, a blank space where adultery had once blared its sordid details. Surely Agnes knew that the real Jezebel (married off to an Israelite king, but with the audacity to bring her own religion in tow—one which allowed women to rule and to celebrate sacred sexuality) came to an equally horrific end. Shoved out of a high window by a rival king, torn apart and devoured by rabid dogs in the street—that was the Jezebel in my Grandma's holy bible. According to those who could read my Gram's martyric tears, she suffered no less.

When it was time, my father drove Agnes to the asylum. That's what it was, he thought; you can nicey it up with hospital talk, but he'd seen how the staff looked down on the patients. He could sense revulsion in the air.

As he drove, Robert Elton thought about special and mysterious burdens. Why couldn't he control this one person in his life? Everyone else bent to his cyclonic will, clamoring for more of his director's eye. At least he could count on his wife, chewing her lip on the front seat beside him.

Especially when Agnes endeavored to make her final statement.

"Are you okay, Mom?" my mother asked. Agnes was too quiet in the back seat. Turning every few seconds to check, Marie saw the pale elder with cheek in hand, staring at the traffic as if it were her life going by. Perhaps she heard it, a ceaseless droning in her head that would not stop: *Die, die, die. Now.*

There were no seat belts in cars then. The click that lifted the lock wasn't warning enough.

So it was that Agnes shifted her weight toward the door and reached for the chrome lever to gritty freedom, her final punishment. She imagined herself rolling along the asphalt like yesterday's newspapers, eating the dust of those who sped by giving nothing but a voyeur's damn, until at last the wheels pounded her, a silenced Jezebel. Did she think about it: how all that was left of the woman in the bible after the dogs finished was her feet, her skull, and her palms lying upturned on the street?

But depression slowed her movements, and youth was quicker. Marie glanced back in time and gasped. She pounced on the woman's sleeve, pulling hard. With all her petite strength, jacked up by adrenalin, my mother wrestled Agnes back to the center of the seat as my father looked for a place to pull over. When she let go, little navy blue threads from Agnes' wool coat streaked my mother's palms.

"There! Sit still! Oh, for heaven's sake, Mom!"

My father held his breath, looking for some harbor off the highway. At that moment, Robert Elton was uncharacteristically left without words—big ones, small ones, meaningful ones. Why pull over? What then? How could he scold her? Who would pay for this? Foot on the brake at the side of the road, he lowered his forehead to the wheel. He felt as though he could not breathe. He would come to know that feeling well. But at that moment (because I remember his driving habits back then) I can imagine the one thought he landed on: *I need a cigarette.*

This was no coffeepot-on-the-toe moment. Mur knew they could not blame each other for yet another suicide attempt—one so potentially gruesome and effective. My mother reminded herself of her duty, because she could not envision life without a husband, even though she was the one tricked into caring for Agnes when others in the family said, *We can't put up with her! You have to take her—oh, Marie's so sweet, she'll do it!* Was she so sweet now? A state of feeling regularly terrified and trapped by Agnes was crafting innocence into a new mistaken identity: I must be guilty of *something* to deserve this.

With one last look of sad resentment towards the back seat, my father straightened, hands gripping the arc of the steering wheel, thumbs flipping like levers sprung. She'd gone too far this time, a lot farther than annoying him with fire and brimstone. Had his mother really meant to fling herself from the car, or was this another stunt like the staged strangulation? Who would he be if she accomplished her own self-destruction? Was it only a matter of time?

Perhaps he sensed the answer in a wife's presence beside him. They formed a united front, just the two of them, melded in horror at the vicissitudes of irrational man. They were certain that no one on their block of new homes with yellow kitchens endured anything like this.

Nor was there any need for the lucky ignorant to know.

Agnes stared at her hands and began to cry. She would not die in the street like Jezebel. Later, my mother would make sure I understood what a first-class martyr could accomplish with tears. Marie Elton slammed down the locks on all the car doors and regarded her mother-in-law with wooden awe. As for the crack in her prince's armor, she knew how thoroughly the man who had no "down home" needed her now—and always would.

But as they sped to the hospital, the nuthouse, the loony bin, the asylum for the mentally unfit, these caregivers of the self-anointed Jezebel each silently turned it over in their own minds: *How much more can we take?*

Chapter 2
THE OTHER FAMILY DISEASE

We were still living in Kentucky the night that big brother and I sat at the table, trudging through supper as one parent disappeared and the other leaned into a greasy sink. Earlier, our father had again mentioned the "interesting person" on his side of the family. "He's either your great-uncle or great-grandfather," he said, then changed the subject. Sam had already researched the deeds of Friedrich Wohler in a library book on chemistry. He thought I should know more about the man.

Across plates of mashed potatoes, my brother whispered, "Out of nothing, he made *piss!*"

Samuel and I were Catholic-school clean, but we'd heard this word from neighborhood kids. I laughed until gravy dripped back out the hatch.

As our mother stabbed at dirty pans with a rubber spatula, Sam tried in his earnest way to explain Wohler's experiments. Had I known that I would someday find myself in the thick of urine samples, with an autistic daughter whose lab tests were many, I would have shrugged with a worldly air. "Pee in a cup, that's the future," I'd have said. Instead, as Sam described how Wohler changed the course of science, I went, "Ewww!"

But Friedrich Wohler never touched anything as yucky as what I imagined that night. He was dealing in white crystalline powder—urea, a waste product of protein metabolism excreted in the urine and other bodily fluids of mammals. Upon creating synthetic urea, quite by accident, he hit the world with this revelation: *You, mere mortal, can also make the stuff of life.* Thus he snubbed Vitalism, the approved doctrine of his day, which held that a "vital force" found only in living tissue was required to synthesize organic compounds. Wohler destroyed that dogma, writing tongue-in-cheek to his mentor, a champion of Vitalism, in 1928:

> I can no longer, as it were, hold back my chemical urine; and I have to let out that I can make urea without needing a kidney, whether of man or dog....

He was twenty-eight years old.

Sam went on and on about other discoveries I couldn't understand, and then our father walked back into the kitchen. He told us about the Elton side, including his own father's deeds as an engineer of office buildings in major cities. How he himself tiptoed on steel beams high in the air as a boy, trailing along behind his dad at the construction site. How the Elton engineer was responsible for the concrete supports that upheld "no less than San Francisco's Golden Gate Bridge!" Our father was swathed in pride over his own sire, and merely ho-hum about the founder of organic chemistry. What of the Wohler genius? With Agnes in the house, there was living proof not of great potential, but of a trend towards the downward slope.

The new land

With Harvard stricken from their vocabulary, my parents' first big break would not be New England. Instead, our destination was provincial, even cowboy: Kansas became the Promised Land, and that was the end of Agnes for us. She was shipped off to live with the youngest of her sons; everyone agreed my parents had done enough. Without her, Robert and Marie Elton were free and clear. I would miss her, but frankly I mourned more for my first and only neighborhood and school. Besides, she was family. I was assured that I'd see her again.

I figured Kansas would be nothing more than a stretch of dry land, but our street was lined with huge, arching elms. Upstairs in our new house were rooms for Sam, Ben, and me. I thought my parents would hate our acquired yokel tint after we'd flirted with Harvard, but they threw themselves into the new place with gusto. Suddenly they were hosting gatherings completely unlike the sedate bridge parties of their madwoman days. Colored lights were screwed into the fixtures, bourbon flowed into 7-Up, and the occasional tipsy colleague wandered into our rooms to chat up the kids.

It seemed that everyone loved my father. The rooms overflowed with company, his favorite drug. Narcissus was in full bloom. Unlike the figure from Greek mythology, my father didn't seek his golden reflection in water, but rather in the eyes of others. Just like Narcissus of the famous tale, he needed an echo to make him whole and was comfortable only with those who held at least a smidgeon of awe in his presence.

The spotlight softened him. Weaving tales of his exploits made him attentive to a drink that needed freshening, a wanderer in the hallway looking for the john. The gaze of colleagues ensconced on his furniture and drinking his whiskey substituted for the happy extended family he'd never known.

And the move offered a fine respite from his difficult daughter, for I hastily turned into someone else in Kansas. My mother said I was surly, and always talking back; she didn't support the rights of teenagers to openly wear the dark clouds of their transitioning. As in Kentucky, I looked outdoors for my haven, although on these shady streets there were no kids whirling by on bikes, yelling and goofing around. Besides, I was too old for that—my next move was junior high. So I walked, and looked, and considered my fate in Kansas.

There was one vacant lot nearby. The neighborhood was old; no one was going to build a house on this blank slate. The lot was not visible from our house and rarely mowed, so weeds grew up along the perimeter to shield this oasis from neighborly eyes. There I sat. I liked it better than stepping into a bunch of two-by-fours and plywood that had been thrown up and sold as a home.

Nature was different in this Kansas place. The new flora and fauna were magical. Buffalo behind chain link fence in the park! Coyotes heard on the edge of town! *Look out for rattlesnakes,* said the rednecks. But most impressive of all were the low rolling Flint Hills, our family's Sunday drive-to spot. I was the only one who found their expanse soul-lifting. My parents sniffed, recalling the tree-packed hills and the racehorses in their paddocks on misty mornings in Kentucky.

I sized up my situation. Raised in a Catholic school and then set down where there wasn't one, I was easily appalled by the belligerence of public school kids. Farming and manufacturing were the norm here, despite the presence of the college campus, partly tolerated. I believed I was unlike any other girl in this new place called Osage End, Kansas. In a burg that size, I would have found her eventually. She, too, would have a fire in her head, a craving to get past the known, the boring, the old—and she would be smart as well.

I was out of sync in other, more visible ways: my accent was Southern, my physique resembled a stick, and I was way taller than any boy my age. So the vacant lot got my vote (at least until I got a stereo). Among all manner of grasses seeking height I sat, thought, and scowled. Or pulled a certain paperback out of my pocket that was my constant companion in those days: *I Never Promised You a Rose Garden*.

My grandmother was removed from the fabric of our days, but she was still so alive in my mind. Though I was yet to comprehend the Wohler Madness, I didn't hesitate to grab Hannah Greene's story of a pubescent girl's schizophrenia off the drugstore shelf in our new hometown. The protagonist was my age when she went bonkers in a particularly poetic kind of way. In the store I carefully studied the book jacket with an unsmiling girl, not gorgeous, not happy. *She is different—I'm different.* With a teenager's simple mind, I turned a key in a rather serious lock.

I was soon disillusioned with being a nobody. The forbidden thrill of public school was quickly overshadowed by the tedium. Trying to adjust to the invisibility and meanness of junior high set me on edge. What others girls prized (cheerleading and crew-cut boyfriends) left me cold. No clues were forthcoming about where I belonged. I tried out various identities through my voracious reading—carefully keeping the more provocative titles about mad girls out of study hall.

It was supposed to be a new life, but I picked up Hannah Greene's book because, even though Agnes was gone, I carried her with me. If anyone asked, I would say that *I Never Promised You a Rose Garden* was science fiction. I didn't know I was searching for why my grandmother went to the nuthouse—or why I'd been so oblivious, and whether or not her kind of trouble was coming for me.

None of my classmates seemed interested in what made people crazy. Yet I understood the protagonist in *I Never Promised You a Rose Garden:* a high school girl who couldn't play the game as school and family dictated. I was fascinated with her vast inner world of fire and sky gods, psychedelic landscapes, and secret language, more real than the so-called real world seen in shades of gray. When the bad guys of Yr (her alternately wondrous and menacing inner haven) spoke in scintillating verse, I wondered if Agnes had ever been this far gone.

Parts of the heroine's schizoform landscape made me envious: she had friends there, and the terrain was always an adventure. As she progressed and gradually said goodbye to Yr, I should have rejoiced. But I sensed a lesson coming from the gray world I woke to day after day.

Just how deep could one hide inside?

Faces I'd rather be

She would come to regret it, but without even trying my mother handed over the ferry that would take me from my misery to a sense of place.

Every month Mur pulled her women's magazines from the mailbox: *McCall's, Redbook, Ladies' Home Journal.* With tips about how to "do for," how to be complete in the gaze of a man, these slick pages were an addiction. Promises to make you gorgeous, popular, and loved were endlessly re-worked. Devour this magazine and learn—that was the message offered by the perky model or pretty mom smiling on the cover of each new issue.

Until one day there was an exception to this wholesome, cover-girl rule. It must have been an editorial risk to forgo the usual Madison Avenue strategy, but in the summer of 1967 there was a hotter topic. One magazine put indoctrination into womanhood on hold to feature row after row of real faces in place of famous ones. They screamed out culture's new fear: *hippies.*

Inside, the writers were troubled. The young faces with unstudied grins stumped them—sons and daughters who should have been in high school or college. The editor pondered why on earth such a large sampling of the nation's adolescents would want to *drop out*. Not just out of school, mind you. Out of expectations altogether.

Because they wanted more than drinking beer and pep rallies, going steady, and death by dull homework? These children were running away to be together, and taking off their clothes along with their parent's values. The magazine used the lexicon *hippies* but the children called themselves *freaks*. Coagulating on either coast, skin painted with neon swirls, smiling too widely for propriety, hair all over the page—they looked at peace, if a little giddy. Clearly, they didn't care who was popular back home.

The article said there was more to their hedonism and grubby clothes than simple defiance. The kids were troubled by competition, prejudice, body counts, and blown-up territory in Southeast Asia. *The problem with you,* the painted faces said to the magazine-as-mouthpiece, *is that you look the other way and let wrong go on. Think you'll ever listen to us? Of course not. So we quit. We quit it all!*

By the time I had digested the article and photographs, I was one of them. Almost overnight I came to care less about school fashions and the sappy fiction inside my mother's magazines. The impact of persons without poses, where no artifice reigned, came like a lightning bolt. I hijacked the issue with those wild faces beaming.

Before long I gave up empire waistlines and sleeping with rollers in my hair. I mouthed new criticisms, wore the wish for another world, and dropped out of the quest for A's and honors at school. It marked the beginning of my end as an Elton, and my father knew it.

Though he saw nothing wrong with social revolt, he felt his daughter slipping out of his control. She seemed reckless, enthralled by ideas that might contain merit but needed refinement. He feared I was gullible and without instincts for danger. At least now he *saw* me, all right. I was no longer invisible! But all I saw was his contempt.

Worst of all, from my father's perspective, I took on the famous Elton superiority. But instead of aligning with the family, once I'd sworn in as a hippie I presumed to be *better than an Elton*.

Everything about the droppers-out looked to me like greener grass. They were leaving the Blah World, these tribes, but they were not insane. They baffled the sedate—but despite all the complaining and focusing on the length of their hair, most adults let them have a go at it. They were kids, and even the Blahs knew deep down that their world had a hole in its soul.

Hippie magazines started showing up at the drugstore with names like *Eye* and *Cheetah* and *Us*. Although each lasted but a few issues, I gathered and treasured those pages. They were full of blatant and beautiful madly sane faces, and daring words of heresy struck like a battering ram at the castles of the orthodox Blahs.

Hip culture lauded elixirs that could take you where it was beautiful to see and to be, minus the pitfalls of Yr. Challenged to do beautiful madness and get away with it, I began to explore chemistry on my own. People like Agnes and the subjects of Yr were captives to time, but my experiments wore off in a few hours. Maybe I had the genes to go the distance, not entirely to schizophrenia, but to somewhere foreign and risky. Drugs seemed like a manageable tour of the outer limits.

By the time I was fourteen, I could pinch myself and know I was real: straight hair in a cascade to my waist, moccasins of soft leather, clothes from thrift stores, illegal baggies stashed about my room. Living on impulse power, I was bound for all the pleasures I'd missed by trying to be teacher's pet and aching to be popular in my new locale. I cemented my standing as school pariah by cutting class to read about mad girls and write poetry in the park.

Kindling for the other family disease

Robert Elton's rage was white-hot. He was angry much of the time—if not at a colleague, for some real or imagined slight, then at me. Our war of words erupted whenever I could not avoid him. My mother said it was because we were so alike.

Why were we all so afraid of him? Because he had been a middleweight boxer, somewhere in the past before children and wife, who still stared mesmerized at "the fights" on TV? Because he turned purple around the neck when his will failed to mow down an opposing argument? Because his temper was no household secret, but was deemed his strength in the teacher's union or, later, in the faculty senate?

Because he boasted that he was a bad ass and made sure to follow up, in one venue or another?

There was no room for two individuals of this stripe in one house. I betrayed Narcissus by setting sights on my own independent thoughts, brimming with opinions, wanting to know who I was. What he needed was readily available energy for his fan club.

"It was the move here that did it," muttered our Mur. With her mother-in-law firmly out of the picture, suddenly she missed Kentucky and didn't care for Kansas. The town of Osage End smelled bad. If the wind blew one way, it was the stink of the slaughterhouses; if it shifted, strange odors from the soybean mill filled the air. She never got used to it. The joy in being free of Agnes proved short-lived when real life closed in—Kansas until retirement! Marie often took to bed, windows closed against the town, with migraines year round and hay fever come spring and fall.

But when she was present, she was as contemptuous and tight-lipped as her man. My embrace of the counterculture swamped her with dismay. How could I go about so untidy? At least, she tried to believe, I would never commit an illegal act. She pronounced my sullen, antisocial, eye-rolling disobedience to be only a hallmark of the teenage times. But those horrible books I brought home—*High Priest* by that drug-peddling Timothy Leary! Those dark and depressing records blaring from my room! Hence my mother and her beloved formed a united front: I was the bad seed. Why couldn't I be more like my brothers? Especially their Number One Son.

❋ ❋ ❋

Sam and I barely spoke. Once I found someone to be, I had no use for him. He became as invisible to me as I had been to everyone else before I grew long hair and wore weird clothes. He had his cherished place as the family brain in mathematics, chemistry, and physics. What I saw as I breezed down the hall, wanting to look into his room, wanting so badly not to, were feet. Toes pointed at the ceiling connected to Sam, flat out and face up on his bed, dirty socks flicking back and forth like windshield wipers.

From the hallway I could hear the racing of his thoughts.

Once in awhile he came down from his room. At the dining room table, homework splayed everywhere, always in white shirt sleeves and worn dress slacks, he sat without really working, his leg continually jiggling up and down, a volcano shaking the floor. I tried to understand beakers and Bunsen burners, but never persevered much past spilling blue fizz all over the Ping-Pong table. Sam had to make sense of it: he was alone with his thirst for things he longed to share.

Perhaps he also noticed I was a girl. *Of course she can't understand!* Yet he kept trying to reach me. Other boys found sports, cars, or stolen porn to captivate them. Sam came early and strong to his subject, but remained unaware of how others would resent this. My indifference to the workings of the universe irked him no end. In his frustration he'd take a swing at that cupola where I should have been racing toward science with all my might. He hit me in the head a lot.

Back in Kentucky, Sam was what polite talk called a "big boy"—he ate and ate as if in a trance. So when a blow came, it was more than a sting. Sam's powerful, pudgy hand slammed against my skull. I yelled, but he had *carte blanche* for the moment. He was the babysitter while our parents were off stalking low prices at the new Louisville mall. Boy, was I ever going to tell.

Punching me for not being touched by his fervor, Sam yelled, "You're not trying!" He had four years on me—and besides, outer space (which I figured this was all about) was a scary place, too big and strange to imagine, like hell. I stared silently and let him ramble, hoping he'd overlook the fact that I wasn't actually there. Forget walking, even running away—not until I'd heard him out, not until he became completely disgusted with me was I allowed to slink off as fast as that stupid-head on my shoulders could steer me.

Back home with their bargains, Marie and Robert Elton sighed as though we'd clashed over choosing a TV program. How to tell them why Sam exploded? The link between his ecstasy over physics and his lashing out was too subtle for me to maneuver. Our parents scowled as if they'd heard it all before, and they had. We were sternly warned, "Cut it out, the both of you."

Writing me off as "just a dumb girl" was Sam's trial run at the prime Elton weapon—contempt—but before long he regarded everyone from inside his armor. He knew he was, as our parents drilled into us, *smarter than the average bear.* But not in the way our literary father had hoped. My brother's thirst for science was admirable, but not interesting to the rest of his family. His circle of friends shrank, and then he found himself in Kansas, alone in a new school with no adult tipped off as to his gift. That's when the midnight screaming in his sleep began.

Ben, the baby brother born just before Kentucky was forsaken, was growing up too. He suffered from continual stomachaches, with dismay in his eyes for his mouthy sister who was always in trouble. He was a bundle of radar in social situations, picking up emotional cross-currents even as a tiny bit of a boy. It was a sensitivity that made him suffer.

I remember when Ben brought home a curious diagram from school, a crude graph drawn by his own hand. Little Brother asked me to take a look. He'd arranged the names of kids in his class in perceived order of importance. The popular kids' names were written large, while the rest decreased in size down to the familiar first names of his two best friends on lower, less fancy rungs. At the very bottom of the page, adrift and apart in tiny script, Ben had written: *me.*

It's not like I wasn't damaged by the peer pecking order. The whole topic was gruesome, any way you looked at it. But wasn't a first-grader too young to be this grim, this hopeless?

Ben played with his car collections and dreamed of his ticket to ride: a driver's license to set him free from the tension, the silence. Already he showed signs of becoming a "car guy." But underneath it all, he was the lost boy in a house full of strangers he helplessly loved.

And then our father broke apart, and everyone was on their own.

From the heart outward

It was the Elton curse, our other family disease: cardiac crisis. Handed down from the Great Engineer, it coupled genetics with a full-steam work ethic, a Type A personality's striving for more. The heart attack was excusable, because it proved you were busting your ass. My dad smoked, drank, and swore his way right into what he knew was stalking him. But my parents' version of the story always held that someone within our ranks pushed him over the edge.

I don't remember precisely when the Heart Problem began. My father's aches and pains gradually crept into our days. Shoulder pain, pain radiating down the arm, chest pain. He made many a pilgrimage looking for The Doctor who would identify his malaise once and for all. Eventually he stole away to the Catholic hospital for tests. His pains were etched onto screens that the experts pondered. A delicate graph spat forth at the end, and at the dinner table my father described each peak and saw-toothed valley of his EKG. Perhaps he dreamed of snatching those clinical papers and bringing them home, slipping them into his file cabinet to burn brightly among the sheaves of literary criticism.

Mostly, Robert Elton tried to figure out what to do about the constant and unremitting pain. Never sure whether to hide or reveal it, he made pronounced rubbing gestures that he dropped with self-conscious speed whenever caught. Wincing as he stretched, flexing his arms as if in supplication, he'd glance bitterly at his audience and then pause, as if stunned into a frieze. After the diagnosis was in, he determined what had caused such a hard-working heart to go bad. Yes, it was genetic, but there was more to it. Agnes had been replaced by another traitor in the house.

My father hadn't given his health much thought while he was striving as fast as he could for all that he could get. He was in his heyday, attacking cherished Kansas figures in articles that the university published, winking at what a bad boy he was. He wished he could have done better than to land in Oz, but once the final version of who was to blame for his cardiac arrest reached the ears of the curious, it turned out that neither town nor career had broken his heart.

How the mighty fall

I was downtown the first time it happened. After school, students emptied into stores two blocks from campus, especially the Woolworth's five-and-dime that dominated the central block. The store both encouraged and despised the young who congregated there in droves, waiting for slim hamburgers on soda-fountain seats that swirled around 360 degrees.

My ritual was to purchase a caramel apple from Woolworth's after school. They were fresh and fabulous, bulbous crunchy things slathered in warm, barely firm goo, balanced on thin Popsicle sticks. It was a trick to eat one delicately—you had to bite it just right, or sticky crud would make fun of your face.

On the first day of many that shook my father to his roots, I was standing in front of the bank with its phony Roman columns, flaunting my love beads to a couple of friends. They were purchased from the head shop around the corner, where a salesman tried to cajole me into the back room for other things. He was a handsome stranger but seemed too grown-up, and my daring was spent simply walking in the door. I had also bought a woven leather headband and was just about to don it, my caramel apple parked in a bemused friend's hand, when Mur pulled into the parking spot right in front of us.

Having your mother drive up that way was the pinprick of deflation. But then suppose she goes so far as to roll down the window, with frowsy abandon, and launch your name into the air. You thought you were so free, so grown up, your friends like converging queens, each with a pocketbook of petty cash. Boys roved in loud packs, arms punching, swift-kicking among themselves to see who tripped. In this setting your mother's transgression shouted out how you were owned.

Mur motioned to me with an arm-sweep that verged on panic. I felt a sudden urge to drop the candied apple, handed over by the friend who was now making fast tracks away with the others. Instead, I carried it like a scepter to the car, where its shine flashed accusingly. As I climbed in and shut the door Marie noticed, without looking, the leather headband that fell onto the seat between us.

"Your dad had a heart attack."

My mother moved as if she would break—not like glass breaks, but like a water-balloon that rips and gushes on impact. The Queen of Tears, her mouth made an unsteady line but she kept jerking her head away. *It's really bad when she tries to hide it.*

"It happened during class."

"He was teaching?" I really didn't know how to feel now. Narcissus holding forth to rows of potential Echos—it was his favorite arena. He was well-liked by students, and I was convinced that there he showed his best side.

Mur nodded. "He had to leave during the middle of a lecture. Then drove himself home." Her admiration for his gall won out over awe at the stupidity of the risk.

In the late afternoon hospital room, my father was cranked to a sitting position, full of zest and jest. He'd been stabilized and was holding court with a number of nurses who stood fingering their clipboards. The white hats parted like a good-natured wave for my mother and me.

"I give 'em a hard time!" Robert Elton chuckled as we entered the room. The nurses rattled their papers as they trickled away, casting back cautions that my father graciously acknowledged.

He peered without his glasses at my tongue-tied stare. "I'm a survivor!" he thundered. "Let's just say I won't 'go gentle into that good night.'" I blinked, dull to the reference, whereupon my father gave a little laugh and looked down at the hospital's cotton shift with its fleur-de-lis print. Wires from under his skin ran to various contraptions.

He then proceeded to dissect every aspect of the operation promised him, but he never spoke about what happened before his students: of bathing in sweat, losing breath, somehow navigating the elevator, hallway, parking lot. I was an expert at going blank when thoughts were unmanageable, and wasn't pressed for comment.

Inside his hospital room Robert Elton assumed the air of a visiting dignitary, second only to one. That would be His Doctor, the greatest man of all, whose worth soared above all others. "I've been all over the country, and this is the only man who can help me," he would say later, after covering many a mile in search of the sage of the moment. My father loved this holy man who dealt in fate with stoic detachment, with the faintest trace of liquor on his evening-rounds breath to show that he was human, after all.

When the visit was over, my mother and I went home, and I kept the dial on mindless. Robert Elton stayed for more tests. He was still under watch at the Catholic hospital when Good Boy called on the phone and asked for me.

Now everyone else knows too

I barely knew the kid. The son of one of my father's colleagues, his call caught me off guard. Good Boy was my age but attended the laboratory school on campus, like Ben and Sam. He was another brain with pens in his plaid shirt pocket and a sallow look about him. Those brainy brats were always kissing up to adults. Had Good Boy and I talked more than once since our family moved to Osage End?

The call came during that post-dinner hour when I pretended to do homework and listened to records instead. Sam commandeered the dining room table and spread his wares conspicuously, intent on working the alchemy of pencil and theorem into the gold of acclaim. It was with half a mind I took the receiver, the other half already tuned to my imminent departure for the stereo to hear *Sergeant Pepper's Lonely Hearts Club Band*.

Good Boy set the tone, and things went fast. "How is he?" the son-of-a-colleague asked.

I mouthed the official report, but neglected to emphasize the wonderful time my father was having, entertaining the hospital staff. Good Boy surely would have responded with an audible frown.

"I want to talk to you about your...dad."

"About...?"

"Couldn't you let up on him a little?"

"Whaddya mean?" I slurred, damned if I'd let on that I knew.

"Come on, what's wrong with wearing a skirt instead of jeans?" (The lab school, I recalled, had a strict dress code.) "And your hair, geez, do you ever comb it? It's a tangled mess!"

Tangled, tangled: my mother's word since childhood for the daily catastrophe that was my awfully thick hair. The word seemed too intimate to be uttered by this guy.

"My hair?" What had happened to the great retorts, the speech of superiority? Run over by the novelty of a sideline-peer who dared to one-up me, I didn't have time to sort out who was the smarter bear.

"And I heard your grades could be better. Listen, we're college professors' kids. I don't know what you're doing at that dumb school anyway."

And your dad's a drunk. Everybody knows it but keeps quiet cause he's such a sweetheart. A perfect retort, and true, but formed only later, far later, after the brat hung up.

All I could think about was how I would never survive in a school where Samuel's contempt could reach me in the hallways. Now here was his proxy, dressing me down to prove it. Initially I had requested to stay in the public school because of my friends. I preferred moving through the simmering pot of blue-collar spawn with a thin upper crust, three floors of brick and mortar perched on the rim of downtown. Seen, perhaps, but not really scrutinized. *No expectations.*

This son of the sodden poet-professor waited for a reply, but nothing snappy came to the surface, nothing to make him pay. My face was warm and my mind held too many floating, unmarked packages.

Good Boy finally wound down. Later, in my room, I shouted: "SANCTIMONIOUS PUNK! PUTRID JERK!" But on the phone I ended only with the line, "Wow, hey, I'll, you know, tell him that you called."

And I did. My father blushed modestly; he said the boy was all heart.

Robert Elton pulled through, again and again, through bypasses and pacemakers and the many scars we were forced to view on his pallid chest. But the walls of the house kept singing *heart patient, heart patient, when will you go?* He began the practice of brooding in the open, beseeching someone to drown with him.

When the Wohler Madness lived with us, there was always an option. Agnes was shipped out. But what happens when the heart attacks? You can't send it packing, or get a new job and leave it behind.

There he sat, brooding with stitches and sutures on a muscle he could no longer will into action.

Professor Elton felt marked, with no hope that the telltale sign would fade. *Disability.* He shifted from a dynamo of magnetic attraction to a lump in an armchair, despairing face pointed at the front door for all to see. I saw a man turning death over and over in his mind. I looked away, and fled. Obsessed with his disease, my father garnered proof of others' reasons to keep their distance. Not only did the Wohler Madness threaten his offspring, but a debilitated core mechanism had also marked him as *weak*. He was a dying man, and the living gave him wide berth.

I still molded my warrior clay after his full-speed-ahead, sometimes-bullying, wily soul. His fire was the antidote to the Wohler Madness: there were those among us *like him*, and then there were the fallen. Just when the categories seemed firm, he fell, too, but differently than the mad Wohlers had fallen. And—this was a privilege—he got to talk about it.

We were constantly drafted into the detailed, blow-by-blow saga of his road to recovery, until one surgery after another failed and there was my father, breathless, back at square one again. He recounted to his colleagues the nuances of medication and microsurgery, the magnanimity of the specialists who split his center wide. The *other* family disease, which befell the Type-A human doing, was admissible in public as legitimate suffering. The man had tried, tried so hard to be a man, but the ticker couldn't take it. Attack, recovery, attack. It was like being a veteran of foreign wars.

But just when you dream of winning a medal for valor, you're suddenly an invalid and people avoid you. Those looks in the eyes of his associates on the proving ground—he read them. Thus ended the parties at our house, as my father studied the growing chasm between himself and everyone else.

My father loved to talk about our family genetics and cardiology at the dinner table. The Wohler Madness remained off limits, however. I feared for our line's double curse, each with its price. Which one was for me? As a hippie-freak, I was sure I'd never work myself to death.

Maybe the only way to sidestep both family diseases was to drop off the conveyor belt of expectations and live by the motto, *if it feels good, do it.* That sounded like sanity to me.

Chapter 3
WHEN THE MADNESS WAS ME

None of us were awake when the Denver police came kicking their way in. Their stomachs growled for lunch but all ten of us slept hard, tuning out the work world beyond our trash-strewn apartment. The year was 1969.

Friends in the back room had a moment's more notice than those who snored directly in the path of regulation boots. The officers kicked the door open, kicked a number of us from our slumber on the floor, and kicked past the rubble to the windows through which the lucky ones had just vanished. Burly and tired and venting age-old grudges, these fathers with their own unruly teenagers collected those of us without IDs.

There was sarcasm at the station when I announced to one and all that I had rights. In no time, Juvenile Hall gulped me down like a little crumb. My Rocky Mountain sojourn was over.

The rule was isolation for the first forty-eight hours. I hadn't spent a minute alone since I left Kansas. Allowed books, I was guardedly content. The decor matched every movie about prisons I'd ever seen, and the girls outside my cell looked scary-mean. Soon the matron on duty came in for a chat and offered me a cigarette—a rare privilege, she let me know.

"Why did you run away from home?"

I would have died there. I had no one. School is a joke and a fascist institution. My parents are hypocrites while the Vietnamese are being blown to bits. Or something like that. These dramatic yet sincere beliefs that passed for an identity were spoken as a mindful representative of my tribe. I had found that tribe in the mountains as a result of my fervent wish never to see the flatlands again, where every moment ticking by seemed to say, "Now! Fling forward!" I had jumped, gone forever from the empty joke of Osage End. I was a runaway, proud to be on the run.

It was all about me and my scruffy brethren sleeping on the floor. Colorado was my choice, my promised land, my hideout. Why would parents thwart my freedom by tracking me down? How could they let me simmer in a juvenile jail? But never did I ask the matron: *How is my father's heart? What have you heard?*

Finally, gently, the matron disclosed the latest Elton plan.

I didn't think twice but only thought, *Yes, anything but a trip back home.* The matron was an intelligent woman, no doubt pursuing some college degree that would take her far from this place. She flexed her kid gloves with the crazy girl that I enacted, using the script I'd come to know as The Descent of the Wohler Madness. The matron was pretty, younger than my mother, self-assured in a way Marie Elton would never be. I wished the matron *were* my mother, wished the matron would work at the mental hospital I was going to, wished she would sit and smoke cigarettes with me and talk the night away. But she left, mulling on how to work the incident into a paper for her night class, and I went back to reading *Catcher in the Rye.*

Soon the dull roar beyond my cell subsided: it was lockdown for the night. I couldn't understand why my dreary cubicle stayed as bright as day. Was I in a different rule-zone than the general population? When my eyelids could take the glare no more I looked in vain for a light switch. The ceiling was miles above me, fluorescents burning fierce under a wire cage. Had my grandmother ever stewed in a room like this one, separated from the others, considered a danger to herself and possibly to them? Through the slim window in the door I peered out through the many crisscross lines. Somewhere, in that dark, was the master control.

Nope, these were no special privileges—clearly I'd been forgotten. No matter, I'd had to read far enough to get my book's hero out of a tight spot. Now I needed to make contact with that finger on the switch. I weighed the consequences of doing something unorthodox, having a hunch that the kind matron had long since gone home.

Beside my bed, another window looked onto the world. Through the iron grate I watched the traffic. From several stories up the little cars seemed to scoot like calm, orderly beetles. I imagined those drivers, free people nosing home to sleep in familiar beds, and tried to reassure myself: *I'm safer in here than on those streets.* The Juvenile Hall was in Five Points, the "bad neighborhood." Then I promptly regretted that thought. It was the first time I'd felt afraid of any place in the city since leaving home. I made a mental note to explore the area with whomever, whenever I got out of wherever.

I was fifteen and fixated on freedom. Tonight, Juvenile Hall was an interesting detour, but really? Leaving the lights on all night? It was rude. Back in bed I fixed the pillow over my head to block the glare. Useless. I would have to raise the dead.

The door was thick and my knuckles made only a puny pop or two. I closed a fist and put more into it. No response. Aiming all I had behind both fists for a quick staccato, it never occurred to me I didn't have the right. It might look like a crazy fit, but hey, I'd play that game just to avoid Osage End, Kansas.

Then came a flash of light on a stick, and the narrow window went bright. In the center was a face with no neck, source of a furious command: "Step back! Let me see your hands!"

I pondered this insult. "Hold up your hands!" she bellowed, and I threw them up like an outlaw captured on *Gunsmoke.* The door opened the width of one massive matron, ready for a fight.

"What do you want?"

I hadn't been yelled at in what felt like a very long time. And frankly, never by a livid stranger as I stood with a perfectly reasonable request on the tip of my tongue. I eked it out, breathless. "The light…I need to sleep."

This matron was another matter. Venom encased her. Her face was cratered; either she hated me, or she hated her job, or she hated everyone in the building. Or, most of all, she hated herself.

"There's no switch in here," I continued with the obvious facts, trying to sound ingratiating as the red face retreated, slamming the door. "Thank you," I yelled, "Sorry for the trouble!" Smarter than the average bear, I tried to be ever so good with the servants.

Imagine having to sit among those silent cages night after night. While the young amazons lay sweeter in their dreams, the matrons only had garish magazines and cheap romance novels to see them through, nothing but print swimming down on coffee. They'd have to breed one hostile thought after another just to keep from nodding off.

Did I feel sorry for her? Yes and no. Had she noticed I was crazy she might have softened a little. She might have had more respect!

Problem was, the light burned on. And on. Every object in the room menaced me as I mulled over this matron's intent. Had she forgotten, again? Clicked the wrong switch, pulling someone else from her dreams when she should have been sending me there? My last card was played. I couldn't take another ray of that wrath. Curling under covers, I tried a paragraph or two and then threw the book on the floor. I was going to cry. I thought, she must not be allowed to torture me, I'm only crazy, and I'm leaving tomorrow!

Just then, the bulb overhead drained itself of blazes and I cried anyway, from sheer relief.

What the Wohler Madness said

Parents, what miracles of restraint you are. Not a telltale line at your eyes, no hint of the martyr in your movements. All that I am you take through this airport calmly, taking me from these mountains to the Great Plains again, that I may dive back into the Family Disease with its singular mantra: *Shame on our genes!*

Today we are a touching sight, the rags I wear blurting my story to passersby, stark against your Sears ensembles. Your perfectly benevolent blankness almost goads me to repentance. I *would* recant, just to have such silent guardians escort me forever through this airport. Never finding our flight, we'd walk eternally on the verge of Going Home.

Your pocket-change rises like a fountain to meet the challenge of my appetite. You watch me lost to food, the one thing you can unmistakably give, received gratefully by this street rat. Voracious from weeks of street living, I eat and eat again: hamburger, fries, my greasy loves. You lock eyes when you think I'm not looking, savoring a sadness together as if I'm not really here.

Bowing my head over a Coca-Cola, I know that later you will sigh over this difficult trial, proof of your unhappy existences. How you will make offerings to your idols: Life Isn't Fair, Life Isn't Perfect, why can't she follow *our* script?

I nursed my answers to unspoken questions: Why can't new shoes, proms, and a boy's ring make me live? Did the novels I discovered on your shelves inspire me? Not even television could destroy this hunger. I was driven beyond your walls because, ever since the days of crazy-martyr grandma and strange-acting brother (not to mention my father's ailing heart) something wasn't right. Outside of our house of paranoia, the world promised more.

I wish I could have seen you, my father, standing before the school board after one of my infractions: taking sacrament in the restroom, the smell of marijuana gripping the sinks, linoleum, and eventually the girls who told. I wish I might have seen that rare performance of the subdued but never groveling parent, a specimen of their intellectual better—how good of you to come down from the alabaster towers tonight. "This mysterious business of parenting," you might have said—and the men in their shirtsleeves may have sat, profoundly thoughtful for one second, before deciding on a lighter sentence for me. The next day I was back in the halls, a puzzle to the hoods whose same acts brought down punishments far more public and severe.

But I am not to be re-admitted to that everyday prison. There is a more serious Bastille waiting me. Your parental neutrality tells me I am flammable stuff—you think me damaged, bad seed bearing fruit at last. Neither of us clearly sees the hand the times have in this, what difficult labor will pass before days of acceptable outrage. It's only a family problem, this disease. I half buy it with the part of me that says I am special, not sick. Soon enough others will find out. Rather than go back to the slow stifle of Osage End, a failed runaway returned to the outlands in disgrace, I'll peacefully embrace this more romantic act: derangement.

The new guerilla in town

I was to be the youngest sacrifice ever among those of us in the running for our family disease. Fifteen and not buying it, I fought diagnosis, confinement, and the destiny that was chosen for me. But first

I had to play along. It was better than a return to the house of hearts broken.

My Bastille had clean glass everywhere and there was light; it wasn't what I expected. Not the overbearing fluorescents of Juvey Hall—this was an all-natural shine. Smiley-faced sunlight, brought in on purpose, the same measured portion in each of the rooms. Novas bursting at the end of the halls, the sun holding court in spacious lobbies. I'd planned for the iron and steel of my grandmother's day, but I was the Eltons' only daughter. They chose the Great Plains Mental Health Habitat because it looked *nice*. There were only four small, rarely mentioned rooms where lockdown was applied for the worst behavior on the wards. At night came the discreet bolting of major doors that led outside, just in case.

Two wings, L-shaped, housed the wards. A bump where they converged, more glass walls facing a bank of friendly vending machines. Then offices, where the daytime elite presided: carpet and manners, all dark and closed up by suppertime.

Shifting between sarcasm and shame, I deliberated during the intake session on who I should be. Walking in the footsteps of my grandmother and all my fallen ancestors, I felt the grandeur of my plight. I was also a grubby runaway who needed to wash her hair. Beside me sat the parental facilitators of this plan, hoping to contain the worst of the Wohler bloodline's tendencies. They tried to maintain their composure while dropping their daughter off at the nuthouse, and succeeded due to all the practice they'd had with Agnes. Cordial as if I'd embarked on a summer-camp stay, Robert and Marie Elton showed no emotion, because cloaking was the art they knew.

Nor could I feel a thing, uncertain in the folds of that same cloak.

Then they left and I realized my parents had indeed dumped me off for someone else to fix. Such was the way when hospitals got involved. There was no more the family members could do.

At least there were a few beards and some long hair among the male staffers. Female aides wore lacquered bouffants and hemlines below the knee; apparently, they had seen the counterculture only on television. Assigned a worker from the pack, it was my luck to be received by one of the tallest and most gentle-mannered of men.

"I'm called 'Bub,' short for Bubba, what my daddy could never quit tagging me with," said the aide who took charge of me. As we walked the long gauntlet of the ward, I stole glances into open rooms. Faces were friendly, questioning. They looked like me, these people. These freaks. A new tribe.

"What's your real name?" I challenged him, grasping for a queenly upper hand as Bub led the way down the hall past the nurse's station, to the end of a ward.

He turned to meet my eye and held it, as if assessing something. "Arkin," he said. "Old last name on my mother's side, lost. Somehow 'Ark' for short never caught on." Waiting to see where all this was going, my aide broke the tie. "I hate Bubba, I tell you what," he laughed, and shared it, just a regular guy.

We stood in my room then. The afternoon had parked its sunniest shine here. I was lucky; it was an end room with a dual bank of windows, and there was no roommate. The doors to the world were around the corner, locked only at night. I would gather the coming visions between four walls alone and breathe the air of freedom near.

Bub nodded at my stuff, pulled out drawers, and opened the closet with the long hands of a languid landlord who'd never have to live here. The room was only plain, not prison-like. Then he replanted the distance between us and went to work.

"Let's go over the rules." He walked me through them as my irritation grew. How could I tell him? *This is no boarding school, no military school, man! This is a haven for the deranged! I will do what I will do because I'm crazy and that will be all, thank you.* I nearly dismissed him mid-stream, but he was cute and that was enough in those days to forestall revolt.

Bub wound up on a pertinent note: don't be late for meals. They won't serve you once the line is done. "In fact, it's time," he said, so we trekked back down the hall and queued up to collect our plates and silverware.

My aide stayed by my side, finding us a table that was empty of eyes and ongoing lives. He spent the meal delicately wiping his short beard, generally unimpressed by my wild tales, runaway blather, and drug talk. Displeasure nicked his brow time and again until I ran out of ways to annoy him.

The food was passable, better than I expected. I surveyed the crowd. Hippies, the vast majority were hippies my age, some older, a great gathering of tribe. Sitting on the outskirts were a half dozen who looked more normal, too normal in fact—like one's parents. There was one other, a wild-eyed boy, probably my junior, hard to tell. Flushed face and mechanical motions, a plain white shirt and shapeless dress slacks. *Keep your eye on that one; he's not tribe material. What is he? And why does he remind me of Sam?*

Longhairs joined us and I made a few friends, acceptance an easy give-and-take. It was like being in Denver, only with restrictions. And how. At least we were well fed—no more panhandling in the park. Then Bub reminded me of the mandatory game in fifteen minutes. No, it was not optional, he said. Get some exercise, he chided, have some fun. "We play volleyball every night."

I laughed, and Bub gave me a quizzical look. When was he going to wise up? I was here for heavier things than the stuff of high school gym class. Volleyball, as my first significant act in this place, was a reminder of everything insipid I'd run away from. I uttered some opposition on principle. *Competitive sports are bad vibes!* One should never do jock things and thereby give a nod of recognition to mere jocks. Bub made it clear there was no choice. With dread I followed the crowd through the doors.

Spring held the evening warm enough for light jackets. Bub was beside me again, prodding me about where to stand. In the crotch of the L made by the conjoining wards was a net on a concrete slab. I shuffled to the edge of the court, visibly pouting. This was preposterous—what does volleyball have to do with madness? If you want to exercise, *you* go exercise; I have deeper waters to immerse myself in. Watching the longhairs, others of my kind, bouncing the ball around proved nothing. *I just got here and frivolity is hardly for Day One.*

It was at the same time too inane and too intimate. Playing like friends, like nothing was "wrong," like we all left our labels back in our rooms. Why did these freaks, my new friends, put up with it? Why weren't we inside discussing the war, or escape?

Besides, I'd been stoned for so long. Roaming streets, thumbing rides, lighting up, awake all night, broke and unwashed. I longed for that month of freedom with a sharp pain as I stared at the net. Bub insisted I take a spot on his team, and without one good reason I was afraid.

Of what? Looking stupid? Flunking gym class? Taller than most females my age, it hadn't been so bad, all those weeks when our teacher shirked lesson plans and yelled "Volleyball again!" But that first night on the court of the Great Plains Mental Health Habitat, I could not move. I stood, head down, defiant, pushing back tears. I thought the whole thing was dumb if not cruel, and I wanted to be allowed that statement.

A scruffy hipster on the other side was set to serve, and I felt cornered by snipers. The ball was a missile whizzing toward others who rose to the occasion with their fists. Eventually it came my way and I literally turned a cold shoulder. As the ball glanced off my head I was humiliated. It reminded me of the whacks given by Sam for my scientific lack of interest. How could they be doing this to me?

Bub lumbered to my side. "Go to your room," he ordered, "You're hurting the game for everyone."

They see my point—*just let me be crazy.* Turning to go, I caught sight of the wild-eyed boy in the white shirt, stepping then retreating in place, scanning the air for incoming artillery.

How mundane the healing temple

Bub knocked and entered momentarily. He had my chart in his hand.

I'd seen him down at the nurses' station, making notes. Judgments I could only imagine, my first impression badly muffed. I knew I couldn't play the personal-freedom card again, the sheer *don't want to!* of the spoiled brat. It was time to launch what I came here to do.

"I don't like balls flying at my face," I told him. "They scare me. Really scare me. Really afraid of it." I was plaintive. *Patient states flying objects make her anxious.*

To my dismay, there was real truth in the words—and it was about more than volleyball. I tried to bluster over it, but certain things, inexplicably, put me into a cold sweat. Like those giant moths that get into the house during summer. Or riding in a car over bridges. The recklessness of sports. Paradoxically, what I called "the world" held no fear: city streets in deep night, hitchhiking highways, hallucinogenic substances, and sex with the next stranger. Bub was trained to call that crazy.

It would be the first time I was able to look through one of The Helpers' eyes. Bub didn't behold the queen in her craziness—he saw the weak, mysterious, downtrodden mental patient. Not the Elton smarter-than-the-average bear, not the angry kid screaming, "Fuck you!" (and I would, repeatedly). The Helpers saw phobia everywhere, as with the elderly patient who was deathly scared of horses, even the mention of horses. Any pointless fear was plain nuts, and that's why, they reasoned, I needed their help.

But I had decided that I didn't. If rules were the extent of their bag of tricks, I was out of here. Schedules and volleyball weren't enough to bring one back from the other side of mind. These people were going to miss the beauty of what I thought I knew, and they were going to pressure me harder than my father on a rage-binge. I'd made a mistake when the adventure sounded less bleak than Juvenile Hall, but surely that was easily rectified. I cinched my poor-me act with Bub, who left to tend the rest of his charges. Then I rummaged for a dime.

A phone booth in the lobby was quiet and comfy for the business of communication. It was wood-worn and especially dark inside. I dialed the Elton house, willing at the moment to call it "home."

It was one thing for Grandma Agnes; maybe she did go to places far worse than this willingly. She had her reasons. Me? I was a kid who happened to be in love with life and hell-bent on adventure. I'd find a way to get back in hot pursuit of that, once I shed this place.

My father answered the phone. He always answered. It was the man's job to broker who-knows-what from who-knows-where, pro or con.

"Hi, it's me." I tried to sound like one of the gang, ready to be picked up from Woolworth's downtown.

"Yes, Sue." Tense, expectant.

"What are you guys doing?"

"We've just had our dinner." I waited for him to ask, *What about you? How's it going? What's it like there?* But the line only hummed with distance. I pretended he'd asked.

"Me too! Huh! Get this. Coerced into volleyball. Some nuthouse! Cheap therapy, right?" I could often enlist my dad in the game of putting other people down. It was the one thing we did well together. But he was guarded, of course, and put upon.

"Well…" He gave me his weak, *whaddya trying to do,* voice.

"Look. This may have been hasty. I don't think this is the place for me. It's not—I don't want to stay."

"But just give it a try." It was a different tactic, that blasé tone again from the airport, the summer camp drop-off with the smiling goodbyes.

"Why can't you understand? It's just a place of rules. It's not right. How do you think this is going to help?" It was no use. I couldn't get him on my side, despite the hatred I knew he held for psychiatry. He had hated shrinks ever since he served his mother up to them, and hated them worse now for their touchy-feely smiles, their beards, their books on what a bad parent he was.

I didn't want to leave the phone booth. As long as I sat there, with one finger hooked into the hole for return change, there was hope. Beyond the booth was the glass bowl of a lobby where anybody and everybody could park their noses right up to the edge, look right in on the crazies sitting with their families, everyone wondering what to say.

What was the message of all that glass? That it's perfectly normal, so have a look? Or you might as well look—crazy folks won't notice your stare? Or, aren't we humane, letting all the light in!

Light will scour madness, or at least brighten the lobby's difficult interactions, the obligatory meeting between the sane and ourselves. Where we can all eat together from the wall of vending machines and be satisfied. "Snacks," the final processed resting-place of all the corn and grain growing in the fields around these grounds, snacks that make us safe with their guarantee of communal logos, their brand names a language we all can speak. United in the glass bowl we can sit for a time, united by food that no person actually touched to make, a universal repast that even the insane can procure for themselves.

My father was about to push me out of the phone booth and into the comfort of those sweet and salty tastes that had ever been my fallback friends.

The slant of prairie sunset painted the lobby's glass with a lavender hue. I peeked out of the booth and saw bright orange crackers, little bags of Sugar Babies, and my next pack of Kools. I saw that I would not wind up sitting in the lobby with my luggage, waiting to be picked up. I could hear my father's breathing over the phone, growing louder, gathering steam that would need to find its way out. I knew I had lost when, despite the fact we were separated by a hundred miles, I felt as if my bones would shatter under the impending blast.

"You're there!" he shouted across the wires. "That is *all* now." Robert Elton had turned to the tactic he knew best, as I always somehow forgot that he would. He was the poor put-upon who should not have to deal with this. He was the professor. The good brain. But pushed too far? He was the fighter in the ring, driven to end it and win.

Not a word about mental illness—he wouldn't stoop to it. Did my parents ever believe it was truly inside of me? Or was I being punished, with a solid cover story? As it was with Agnes, so shall it be with one or more from the next batch, the generation up and coming. These things are our destiny.

A bad seed, a crazy mind, what was the difference? You put them somewhere, some place where they wouldn't bother you for a while, maybe never again. Then you grieve—not so much because you miss the person, but because the whole weird twist of fate gets raked over repeatedly by friends and acquaintances catching the gossip on the fly. My parents saw themselves as tragic figures of epic proportions.

"We'll see you next weekend," my father said coldly, and ended the call. Why go on? He held all the cards, or rather the only card that mattered: health insurance.

I always backed down. For the moment.

When my father got angry, it now possessed a special meaning for our family. If he reached up to grab a shoulder, then I was a villain if I continued to speak another word. They'd seen to it that I knew who was responsible. Which was why I ran away: between my father and me, one of us had to go.

Had I caused one more heart attack, this time it would be his end.

There, matron, now you have the real story.

Crazy goo

I rose in the middle of that first night, a mental hospital patient remembering this was war, and it was my move.

Aides, nurses, how promising your titles seem. At last, am I to find the ones who truly assist? Alone in a bland room in the hours of the wee a.m., may I put back nonsense onto floors too cold?

My real tribe, my freaks of a feather, fellow loons inside of here or on the street: we often made ourselves high by operating on whim. Surely I hooted out loud when I got the idea about how to get the Blah World's goat, since it thrived inside this place, the proxy of peaceful sleepers in Osage End, Kansas. Someone had won only the first round in the phone booth. The fight would go on.

Foraging among what little hipster paraphernalia was allowed to me, I found two pots of Day-Glo paint, orange and green. A little brush to wield the colors, a brush too demure for blank walls. These walls were calling out for my paint, but they would never get enough. I thumbed my nose at them and went over to my toiletries.

A simple tube of toothpaste, pristine white. But what a soft long skinny snake body it made as it oozed onto the floor, guided by the groove between the frigid tiles.

Now for the finish. Two squeezes of Pepsodent fanning out from the tip made an arrow pointing to freedom: the door. But that white arrow gelling between the beds called for more! I invoked the black-light aura of any respectable Denver crash pad and set to work with orange and green.

Will you aid me, Helpers, will you nurse this hand that unscrews the caps and dips into colors best seen under the effects of herbs that horrify you? Will you find hideous the hues that I weave in short squiggles and stripes, or will you suddenly find truth? I could step around this floorshow for days—won't you also honor consecrated ground?

At last the arrow, dotted and swiped with happy color, meant that I could sleep again. Tit had been exchanged for tat. I'd made my point: the arrow ran from beside my bed, straight to the door. *I am here.*

But I will not be for long.

When morning came, it was clear that my message flopped. The unlucky aide on wake-up rounds stopped short of getting tooth-paste on her patent leather pumps, and called for backup. None were charmed. I tried to soothe them with a rant on freedom that fell flatter than my floor art. I prayed they'd find me only messy and forget the whole thing, but a deepening crease on the brow of the head nurse did not bode well.

Fine arrow, pointing to no real point, I fear these are your last seconds. Now we know, don't we? I came here for succor, that's why I agreed. I came here to dive into all I am and dance with it, and then be seen. I came here because Agnes Wohler Elton walked a similar line, though she didn't paint one like this. I have to know how she skirted it. Yet all the Helpers misunderstand you, dear arrow, they take you for mere goo. Now they huddle, and haggle over consequences, and I'm the sitting duck.

In came the cleaning supplies. The aides grumbled under their breath about salaries that weren't worth it. So they handed the mop to me and I took it up, under force, registering complaint the Elton way: snide and personal, so you feel the sting.

But something else was offered alongside the disinfectant: a little paper cup in the hand of one determined nurse, extending right-angle from her body, elbow propped as if she could hardly bear her life. I looked in as if I didn't know that there were pills in there.

"These aren't my sacraments," I told her.

"Well, these are your meds."

I could tell she thought I wasn't myself—as if she knew. They all pretended to look through me, especially if they had kids my age—and damn it to hell, they all did.

"This will help," said the nurse, referring to those petite round deceivers with a company name inscribed in flowing scroll.

"Leave them here, then," I wheedled, "I'll get to it after cleanup." *Then maybe you will forget, because I am not going into that colorless haze, and that's that.*

Perhaps because it was only my second day, perhaps because the Day-Glo goo couldn't sit another minute in her sight, the nurse let it go. I could feel, though, how much she wanted that little cup with its pharmaceutical mysteries to become a frequent visitor to my room.

So. This is the way that Agnes went.

Not only with a shock, but also a swallow.

Entrenched, ennui

After six months in the Habitat, a not-so subtle pressure began. I was getting too comfortable. I was settling into institutional life. In my mind, I could have lived there forever. But the insurance money was running out, and my parents wanted me back home.

I had run short of ways to bug the staff, whose preference was to ignore me. Their new intensity was focused on neither my thoughts nor my feelings, but rather on my need to start exhibiting more toe-the-line behaviors. Like *wanting* to go home. With the handwriting on the wall, I figured I should try everything the place had to offer, just because—and just in case I was whisked back to Osage End.

The phrase *substance abuse* did not exist in 1969. Nor, for someone thin as a rail who starved herself between binges on sugar and starch, was there such a thing as *eating disorder*. The front office fell in line with the expectations of the Wohler Madness and christened me *paranoid schizophrenic*. It felt ponderous, important, and somehow a tribute to my grandmother. But I also had a sense of being ripped off: I wanted the immediacy and the colors of Yr. Inside, I knew I was only unloved, and unlovable—and that's what everybody missed.

Daily I had to get outdoors, to the edge of the grounds, or I would feel choked by the disapproval of the parental stand-ins, under the gun by health insurance running swiftly through the hourglass of time. A low-security facility on a rolling piece of prairie meant no fences, locked gates, or permission needed to stroll. The Habitat turf ended where acres of wheat began, so I walked into the field and sprawled there, golden spires ringing my hidey-hole. I could have laid low and made the staff come find me, but why? The field was freely available, and back inside the food was pretty good.

Sometimes I went behind the cedar tree, tall and spreading like a woman in petticoats, just ten yards from my room. There, one could neither see nor be seen by the wards. Sprung momentarily from the nuthouse culture I would relax with cedar, wheat, or sunset, because these things all told me it would turn out to my satisfaction in the end. A lonely teenager, I sought nature to soften the effect of the constant frowns and sarcasm that came my way. But still I waited for human faces to define me. How could a flouncing cedar do the job?

At least if I couldn't climb one notch above the average bear any other way, a stint in the loony bin would surely count. What would they think back in Osage End, that hateful place I never wanted to see again?

The color of time wasted

I remembered laughing when an Okie uncle on my mother's side suggested I had a drug problem. What fifteen-year old wouldn't want to be high all day, charging into sub-worlds peopled with veteran addicts who were suffering serious soul loss? I called it getting down with the people—*real life!* The Great Plains Mental Health Habitat knew better. Its influx of adolescents revealed dangerous mental illness in the young—our penchant for grass and acid was merely the telling sign of our disease. It was nuts to act like a hippie and our parents, of course, would pay any price to have the urge removed.

Few of our tribe cared for "downers," but they were the Habitat's drugs of choice and plentiful for the asking. The staff didn't consider us violent (we weren't), just smart asses (we were). A brisk, clandestine trade in palmed meds meant Thorazine reigned as the king of the downers. I wondered if I was missing anything by steering clear. Eventually, I traded a favorite record album for some stockpiled Thorazine, just to see what it did to my head.

The morning of this experiment, I let my close friends know. What I didn't know was squat about dosage or "side effects." If this was really something special, one couldn't take too many. I swallowed all the Thorazine that a freckled, red-haired boy on the edge of our tribe handed me.

And went to sleep for hours, far into the afternoon.

It was a weekend, so there was no scheduled round of therapy and busy work. I missed lunch to no fanfare. When dinnertime loomed, my confidantes tried to wake me. "You have to come eat," they urged, "or they will *know* about this." They managed me to my feet and dragged me to the door.

It was summer, a real scorcher of a day outside, and I could feel them anxiously pulling on my bare arms. Yet when I looked out the glass doors toward my beloved cedar, things did not compute.

"Is it snowing?" I asked.

Outside, everything was white, pure white—even the sky. Pharmaceutical white.

Somehow I managed to walk, grab a plate, and fake my way through the mess hall ritual. At the table there wasn't much to say even to my best friends in the whole world. My face felt like modeling clay. None of us smiled; they were tensely watching to see who might be watching me. The food was tasteless and I worked hard not to droop. I would have puddled up in a heap of hair, flesh, and bones all over my plate had it not been for the banter that aimed to include me every other minute. My best friend bussed my dishes while I made the supreme effort to cross one leg over the other and smoke the usual cigarette.

Flanked by be-bopping escorts who tried to draw attention away from me, I made it back to my room. My friends fled. No fun in watching me snore.

"Just really tired today," I told the nurse who looked in, and frankly preferred this to my usual acting out.

None of our keepers suspected a thing. It was nice to have me quiet on their shift for a change, on that day when I could have died.

Chapter 4
MAD WORLD

For Chris Glen, "fear of flying" was an understatement. We were still on the ground but he'd already waylaid the stewardess three times, asking about weather conditions, the safety of the plane, and the crew's track record in risky situations. Chris was my husband—an older man, age twenty, carting off "sweet sixteen."

I was finally, ecstatically, free: from the Habitat, from Kansas, from the house of cardiac crisis, from the brothers who played Good Kids opposite my role as Problem Child. Our plane would be in the air for four hours, destination San Francisco.

Chris was a counterculture dream come true. We met when our family visited the Finley farm in Oklahoma and a cousin introduced us at the home of some local freaks. Chris produced his calling card of bulging baggies from his Army surplus pockets. "You want acid? You want pot? Speed?" Days later he came to Osage End at my request, and stayed. A drifter, he was stalled—but his resume was impressive. While chapter head of Students for a Democratic Society (SDS) at a California state university, he'd smoked dope with the likes of Black Panther Bobby Seale and SDS's Tom Hayden. He'd marched, he'd raged against the Establishment, and he hated President Richard Nixon with a passion.

After hitchhiking to Osage End and installing himself in a deserted crash pad near the college, Chris' first task was to educate me. The books he slid toward my willing mind were gobbled up like hard candy—difficult to break, but sweet with satisfaction. Eldridge Cleaver, the serious Marx brother Karl, China's Chairman Mao, and poems by Vietnam's rebel leader, Ho Chi Minh. I whipped them out proudly during study hall, and made sure a revolutionary tract was on top of the book stack I lugged from class to class.

My beau's message was four-part, and during our strange courtship Chris Glen drove it home continually. The war was wrong (we agreed); socialism was the only way (I could see that); armed struggle was necessary, especially if it was waged by the vanguard (which we were).

"Guns," he concluded, simply.

I laughed at him. "You mean, as in *bang-bang*?"

But I wanted to be loved.

Chris never owned a gun, never held one, let alone pulled a trigger. When we finally landed in San Francisco, after much histrionics and stomach-calming ginger ale, there was only his very straight-laced sister and her mortician-fiancée to greet us. His fellow revolutionaries were nowhere in sight.

Why did my parents allow their under-age daughter such a grown-up commitment at the age of sixteen? They were weary, I guess. "We didn't think we could stop you," they said. Thus the Eltons struck a sympathetic chord among their colleagues, who felt helpless before teenagers they construed as pulling the strings. By the time Chris sat at our dinner table, my parents had already shown me how far they would go in considering me the heiress to the Wohler Madness. We never discussed my time at the Habitat.

But what I regret is the loss, over the decades, of the essential points of the Elton arguments. All that remains is the simplistic, infuriating stuff: *Cut your hair, don't wear Salvation Army muumuus, take those moccasins off your feet, don't smoke cigarettes, you're not staying out tonight.* I long to reconstruct the rationales, the philosophical course of our disagreement. The two of them were long-winded, and frequently I had no retort. There was no desire on my part at the time except to erase the words immediately, fearful of what would follow when my father had had enough. I wished for a benevolent Yr to put between myself and them.

Outside the house I adopted the tactics of an ultra-sneak, fretting constantly about getting caught. Somehow, settling for the limited options in the Elton house—meek (brothers) or rageful (parents)—felt like getting closer to the sinkhole of the Wohler Madness, a despair so deep that the further one fell, the more paralysis of the will set in.

That is, until Chris Glen came pulling on my heartstrings. He was my ticket beyond a repetition of the timeworn script.

When my parents accepted the inevitability of becoming in-laws, I felt I'd gotten away with the ultimate coup. Upon our engagement, they offered to let Chris sleep on the sofa bed in our house. He cut an interesting figure at the evening meal: wiry and no taller than me, his hair was perilously charged, standing out from his head in a scrawny mane. His eyes darted as a matter of course, his movements jerky when trying to be a helpful guy, languid when on the defensive. We all talked about the Vietnam War and police brutality over pork chops and iced tea.

Chris had a pressing problem. He enlisted my father's literary bent in an endeavor that was bound to fail. To avoid being harvested for the war effort, he wanted to go "CO" (Conscientious Objector), and needed to present his case through a persuasive essay. Trouble was, he wasn't willing to portray himself as a man of peace.

Chris urged "revolution" in every sentence. His heroes all used the barrel of a gun to effect change. He had a flair for slogans ("Off the pigs" was a favorite). "Pigs" were his word for the police, little broken off pieces of President Nixon himself.

My father tried to explain the necessary logic behind going CO: a total, no-exceptions commitment to nonviolence. He was calm and diplomatic, as with a difficult student, and it was like tasting a slice of the forbidden fruit: the professor we never saw in action. But in the end, the in-law-to-be washed his hands of Chris.

And continued to watch the nightly news in dismay. My father gasped at cops out of control, and felt personally assaulted by the Kent State killings, students shot down on a small campus like his own. But he could not visualize his only daughter as part of the picture, and he could hardly support battalions of rag-tags like Chris Glen playing with guns. Besides, the government's instructions were clear. Conscientious Objector meant a belief in *no killing: no exceptions*. Chris wanted to bend the wording. In the end Chris wrote it his way, and was denied CO status.

So our wedding day was a hippie guitar ceremony inside the El-ton living room. My parents would not consent to the neighbors' eyes prying into the backyard celebration we had requested. For the photos, however, Chris and I charged into the front yard. An American flag hung next door and we posed in front of it, he with an angry scowl and raised fist, me with a happy grinning peace sign.

My parents were unreadable on the way to the airport. Not that we were watching them. Kissing and tickling in the back seat, I staunched my terror of the unknown with *I can't believe it's true*. The dream was nigh: San Francisco. I'd poured over pictures of Haight Asbury and the Golden Gate Bridge, the hills, the cable cars—a land unlike prairie in every way. All I wanted was to stop offering my hippie-girl parody to a small town not amused—or worse, not even noticing. To live near San Francisco was to settle into the center of a creative tableau and let it re-make me in its image. To The City I offered myself as a blank slate.

But on the plane, my new *husband* (we both had trouble with the word) had a bomb to explode between us.

"It's best," he began—I expected a treatise on some new aspect of revolution, some future blueprint for a socialist paradise—"if we go straight now."

Straight, back then, meant no drugs, no alcohol, no highs. *Straight and narrow*. I howled with laughter. The flight crew probably registered relief that Chris was being entertained away from his anxieties about air travel.

But my humor was short-lived. My husband was all too willing to step into the shoes of Chancellor Dad. Just when I looked forward to the more intoxicating aspects of adulthood, the groom grounded the vehicle of my rebirth. Without weed, acid, speed, or even alcohol, I'd never become a true citizen of San Francisco. What a double cross!

Where he found this mandate was never clear to me. There was no requirement in the revolution to teetotal. Inebriants were the spoils of our guerilla war. It was the first of a number of heavy-handed moves thrust upon a Kansas kid without a home, and Chris took to their enforcement as if he had inherited the knack from his Navy sergeant father.

Once we settled into domestic life, he checked the odometer of our car to monitor my movements, forbade me to keep company with new friends, and rifled through my belongings for clues to transgressions. The honeymoon was over in a hurry. I would never forgive him.

Had I traded one jailer for another? Did I feel betrayed? Yes and no. I felt like it was all my fault for never, ever seeing it coming. But all that was later. I was sixteen! This was love! This was also California, a long way from home. I felt stuck with Chris, too scared to leave because I didn't know how to navigate on my own. I was too afraid of going home and admitting defeat.

Chris was a radical, so maybe he was right about the ill effects of being high. But what were we doing instead? He became increasingly obsessed with rock and roll stars, and less so with revolutionary theorists. I was waiting to be inducted into his cadre, but the cadre never existed. All said and done, Chris was essentially a loner.

Well, I knew how to write my jailers off. How to rebel without getting caught, how to give a semblance of compliance while seething and biding one's time. Was Chris Glen intent on bumming my trip? I believed he was. Did this kill love? Oh, yes it did. But was it familiar? Even doable? I guessed so.

Chris had a job, which was the one condition my father had placed on the wedding going forward. While my husband worked, I read and thought. Growing up with my suicidal grandmother and schizophrenic brother prompted a need to make sense of the mind-suffering around me, amplified in a world torn over the Vietnam War and civil rights. Married, but still waiting for my senior year of high school to start, the rhetoric of revolution made everything clear. The nuclear family was bourgeois, and it was all the better to put distance between me and mine back in Kansas. Worse than demonic Republicans, soft liberals the likes of my parents were wishy-washy fence sitters. Small towns were counter-productive places for our kind, the vanguard. On the coast we were poised to overhaul the nation.

I focused on how to be a revolutionary, giving little thought to the irony that Chris worked at a state psychiatric hospital practically across the street from our apartment. It might have been the kind of place where Agnes outran her grief, but I had decided that the Wohler Madness was too bourgeois to bother with. As an aide trainee, Chris was groomed to work with the hard core, the true crazies. They had little to do with me, I reasoned, looking back on the Habitat stay where hipped out runaways and desperate housewives had filled the ranks. Besides, with the imminent overthrow of America, all inmates would soon be free.

Then came the suggestion that madness itself was an act of revolution.

Rebels of mind

California offered plenty to digest at face value. Leather-jacketed Black Panthers advocating violent overthrow of a racist government hawked their newspapers on the sidewalks next to unsmiling, crew-cut Socialist Workers with their own publications in arms. Down the block, Hare Krishnas chanted and swirled in orange robes, heads shaved, begging for money through ecstatic dance. Chris' stint as a psych-tech never lasted past the trainee stage; he continually challenged and ignored the higher-ups, whom he called fascists. We were on the move a great deal, and finally found ourselves living with his revolutionary friends from college.

Five of us squeezed into an apartment in East San Jose, where the locals were friendly. *Viva Aztlan!* ("Long Live Our Aztec Homeland!") read the graffiti on the walls, but it was too early for most residents to care about keeping Whitey out—and very few of Whitey wanted in. Chris' friends, three brothers from a "nice" family like mine, were "organizing" in the neighborhood. The neighbors ranged from neutral to supportive of our efforts to kick our privileged roots in the teeth.

Boogie was the youngest and most freewheeling of our three roommates, and secretly I nursed a crush on him. It pained me not because it seemed like emotional infidelity, but because Chris had convinced me I'd never be good enough for someone like Boogie. With spiraling curls down his back and a friendly, carefree manner towards all, he was a psychology student at San Jose State. His brothers fondly teased him about this "revisionist" pursuit. The older two also combined derision and affection when they called him a hippie, a stance they found self-indulgent. Yet while Boogie did his part against the war and touted the armed struggle creed, he looked at things differently.

"Here's something for you," Boogie announced one afternoon, breezing into the apartment with a stack of textbooks and a strange little paperback. He'd knock off classes early, touch base in the apartment, then embark on private odysseys—part socializing, part organizing. I always tried to be somewhere near the door when he got home.

The paperback slid from the pile and Boogie caught it before it smacked the floor. He tossed the thing toward my guarded demeanor, all angles and fringe, parked on the couch.

It was the first time I'd made it so clearly onto his radar. My hands shook with the enormity of that in light of my crush, but I pretended to be skeptical and held the projectile at arms length. The cover of the book was jet black with a mandala of psychedelic images in the center, right under the title *The Politics of Experience*.

"Some Scottish guy—a shrink, but don't let that scare you," said Boogie. "He's the shrink you need"—then, seeing my wary eye, he continued—"that we *all* need. To unshrink us. Trust me, he'll inspire you."

"What's this got to do with the revolution?" I demanded.

Boogie hooted. "Everything! You mentioned something about your family disease. You've got to hear what this doctor thinks about people who go mad."

I was swooning—I was seen! But did he think I was nuts? Boogie went about his usual pit stop and left for the evening. The minute he walked out, I turned expectantly to the words of R.D. Laing and tore through the book, recognition and gratitude dawning as the chapters mounted. Eureka! I knew there was more to madness than volleyball and following the rules!

When Chris returned from job-hunting (or more likely from his haunt of used record stores), I didn't look up. I wanted to be well versed in Mr. Laing before Boogie came back from his night of catting around.

The next day we were all in the apartment, bored and lolling. Boogie's older brothers, Brett and Barry, were reading the Sunday paper and commenting on the revisionist running-dog media's portrayal of events. Baby brother emerged from his room around noon, after a healthy night of party and rhetoric. Chris was cooking, a recent hobby of his that drove Brett and Barry up a wall, because they felt it took his attention away from more serious matters. When Boogie sat down to taste the results, I saw my chance.

"R.D. Laing," I mused. "If only he could run every nuthouse in the world."

"There would be no nuthouses," Boogie quipped.

"Can't have all the crazy people running loose, though?" I remarked sarcastically.

Chris butted in with this observation: "If Nixon is considered sane, we are all in trouble." He had a need to commandeer the conversation, and this parallel track was his best shot. But Boogie and I had a link.

"He doesn't say anything about the war, this Mr. Laing," I challenged Boogie.

The psychology major rose to address his topic. "He'd probably say it's the ultimate madness. He thinks the stifling of our really, truly felt experience is like a war on each person in this society. That kind of thinking rose out of the whole concern with 'alienation'—and Laing credits that. Alienation—guys were talking about that in the fifties. The *Leave It to Beaver* days—when every person on the block was supposedly content, and obedient."

I thought about Kentucky. I was content in my ignorance of the Wohler Madness as it afflicted my grandmother. I was obedient in Catholic school, willing to absorb the tensions and rage of my parents as part of the deal. Out loud, I reflected that Laing's views were published the year my parents started wondering if I were a chip off Agnes' block. Did mental hospital staff read R.D. Laing?

Boogie flipped a mass of curls off one shoulder and prepared to dig into Chris' latest omelet. "Are you kidding? Like they want to believe that any of the so-called patients might be having an experience of value? Laing says that just because the psychiatrist is out of contact with the patient, it doesn't show there's something wrong with the patient—but with *him*. Could mental hospital staff believe there was something *wrong* with *them*?"

I had to agree; I knew from experience. "Patients are bad and mad. Wrong just by being sick in the head."

"Right," said Boogie through a mouthful of food. "They represent the void. Laing would say asylum workers are missing out on what the patients have to teach them."

By now Brett and Barry were listening in. "You mean a crazy person can teach me about politics, economics, how to organize in this neighborhood? Right." This was Barry, the leader of San Jose's Liberation Front, with the editorial section of the newspaper scrunched in his one good hand. The other hand, as usual, was tucked out of sight.

"Yeah," the younger brother replied, "but maybe only as an example. The idea is that there's something essential about going crazy. Laing and others talk about it as a voyage, a journey, even a natural process. I think Laing calls schizophrenia 'exploring the inner space and time of consciousness.'"

"Ha!" erupted Barry, "don't you do that every night with your loco weed?"

"Sometimes. If I wanna. But I still get up, go to classes, and look like a normal alienated automaton," replied Boogie.

I wanted to say, *But you're not! You're sweet, you're caring! You're spending your morning talking to me!*

Chris was standing at the sink, his arms crossed. "I don't know, I just think you have to put up a fight against the powers that control the wards," he said. "I tried working in those prisons for the...ones on the journey."

"So when are you ever going to get another job and stop baking cookies?" asked Barry. Chris ignored him.

Brett, as always, diffused the situation. He was the calm twin who played off Barry's fire. "Szasz is the one they made us read," he commented, long thin arms akimbo on his knees, leaning up to address the kitchen talkers. Brett had been a sociology major once, but worked now with those he and Barry called the "lumpenproletariat," the lowest of the low in terms of socio-economic class. These were the unemployed, the infirm, an "unproductive" rung beneath the blue-collared world. Brett hoped his younger brother would find more meaningful work than his own cubicle inside what was called, without euphemism, the Welfare Office.

"Thomas Szasz. Now there's a mind," Brett went on. "Talk about ahead of his time—Sue, he published *The Myth of Mental Illness* in 1960. But he started congealing all his ideas for the book," Brett's hands stirred the air into an imaginary ball, "when you were one year old. Now *that's* bucking the system."

"All right, so what's he say?" asked Boogie.

"Just that there is no such thing as crazy people, only human problems like anger, despair, loneliness—and that what we call therapy used to be the business of moral philosophy, no stigma attached. Nothing empirical about it. It wasn't science, it was…well, it was philosophy!"

"Right," interjected Barry. "Marxism, Maoism, they're all philosophy. How they're applied, that's our job."

Brett looked uncomfortable. "Well, Dr. Szasz has as little use for Marx as he does for Freud, but that's his opinion. What he says about warehousing the mentally ill is totally right on. In our so-called civilized world they're the unwanted, the troublemakers. That's how it's always been—if you look back into the last few centuries, the poor were the insane. The insane were always poor."

If Boogie was my crush, Brett was my favorite, the most comfortable person in the house to be around. He was a big scarecrow of a guy, but always fair and easy in temperament. His perennial shirt-sleeves and khaki slacks were an effort to remain uncategorized, a blank slate for the unfortunate who dragged their woes into his tiny cubicle, wheedling for more money or time. I listened to him more than the other two, so I asked him how to spell the doc-author's name and what the title was, again.

I loved these guys! Where would I ever find conversations like this in Kansas? But Barry, Mr. Revolutionary, was not amused. "Boogs, give me a break, man; don't tell me that nutballs are explorers. There's no time for such nonsense. Man, the pigs are about to kill us all, the military's on a rampage against a tiny, defenseless nation, and black people are fighting for basic rights every day. Don't give me this 'inner world' crap!"

"So what do you think crazy people should be doing?" I asked Barry. The silence that followed was the result of collective surprise.

Sue rarely spoke to Barry; she didn't know how. Everyone in the apartment knew that he could demolish her with his logic, rhetoric, and grasp of history. Normally I *was* timid and tongue-tied with this ultimate revolutionary, the mastermind behind the San Jose Liberation Front, but the question spilled out before I had a chance to think. Even Chris looked uneasy, but everyone wanted to hear Barry's take on this one. Maybe he'd be kind.

"The mental patients need to organize! Whaddya think? Best thing for getting your head together. You can sit around and mope, or you can fight the power. Chris, man, that omelet smells great—but when are you going to help us out here? We've got a Tenants Union in the works, we need to get the city mobilized for Nixon's visit, I'm up to my ass copying the latest flyers about our platform. What's with you, anyway?"

Everybody knew what was going on with Chris, and everyone but Barry was willing to leave it alone. Barry's job, since he could not work, was organizing San Jose, plus any points beyond he had time to reach. Barry had *overcome* in a very big way.

I stole yet another of many looks at Barry's bad arm. A touch of cerebral palsy had shriveled it at birth; it hung at his side, the hand a small claw that Barry often kept tucked inside a too-long sleeve. He was only a slightly sturdier version of his twin, but wore denim and black leather to give him a tougher, "working class" look. He beamed when the workers he leafleted outside of factories assumed that he mangled his arm in an industrial accident.

Barry didn't need to work; he was cared for by trusts set up by the boys' bourgeois parents. He felt it was his duty to be useful, and quickly assumed leadership among his peers. They were all too happy to let him have it, and the kind of respect he garnered wasn't pity for his bum arm. If anything, the disability made him more of a badass, for Barry was the kind of revolutionary we all wanted to be, but could not bring ourselves. Chris and I used to whisper that we were glad Barry was on our side, instead of a grand wizard in the KKK or a close aide to Tricky Dick.

I too kept waiting for Chris to get "involved"—so that I could. He was partly distracted by job-hunting, by our fights, and by his record collection. But it was clear that there was no place here for Chris to shine. This was Barry's turf, and Chris was not about to play second fiddle. So he cooked, and set himself the task of monitoring my thoughts and movements. He was driving me as crazy as my father did on one of his contemptuous streaks, and my fantasies about running away surfaced again.

Then floundered. Where would I go?

Adrenalin for the antidote

Each exit from our apartment into the city confounded me with an ominous sight on the horizon. The hills in the distance wore a dirty cloak that often hid their curves completely. Smog—the year was 1970, and it was a fascinating horror for a Kansas girl to see trouble in the air she breathed.

Crimes were being committed against the natural world, but my cohorts in revolution considered environmentalism a sissy thing. The killing of the Vietnamese, the epidemic of racism, and the plight of the workers was our focus, for overthrow of the government was nigh. Then the polluting would stop as a matter of course—once we were in charge. I slowly learned to accept smog as a dark reminder of the heartless military-industrial complex.

Nature in the city was accessed by escape—we packed into someone's old car and headed beyond the bustle, up Skyline Drive into the hills. What did we do there? Just sat. The beauty was breathtaking, the filth of city air from a distance like a drab sheet draped over toy buildings. Sometimes the B-brothers brought out flattened cardboard boxes and we climbed aboard, roaring down the dry grass to a gulch below. It was a rush.

With one more year to complete before my diploma, I headed into the smoggy foothills to suburbs that were nothing like back home. Bussing out to the high school was an eye-opener. Along the perimeter of its angled pods the entire complex was wrapped in cyclone fence. Students were not even allowed access to the parking lot on their lunch hour. There was no cozy downtown next to this new school, no quaint caramel apples for sale. And unlike the other students, I had no parents waiting just beyond that high wire fence.

Still, I felt time wasting. I so wanted to please the B-Brothers, and what Barry said about organizing as a way to heal the pain of Crazy (which of course I was not, but just in case) made sense. Inside this high school, I wasn't the only eccentric. There were plenty of bad girls smoking in the bathroom. I had to distinguish myself somehow, and the conclusion was foregone. The three brothers at home put me up to it. *Strike!*

At first Barry didn't find high school relevant enough to coach me, but my desperation to be one of the revolutionaries made him relent. He loaned me one of his underlings, barely past graduation day himself, to strategize the plan.

The war in Vietnam was escalating while American college students died on campus pavements for expressing dissent. The least I could do was wear a black armband, hand out the same at every opportunity, and promote the idea of a walkout against the war.

Due to our confinement, there was ample time to work the crowd. Lunch recess was spent on the grounds. My peers stretched out on green spaces or sat at concrete picnic tables, awash in a stoned haze, sneaking cigarettes under cover, backbiting and sniping. A friend of the B-Brothers gave me a script to improvise on—one that appealed to the massive ennui of those who knew they were stagnating inside this cage.

It didn't take long: one day I planted the seed and the roots spread quickly through the lolling crowd. First a significant number stood up to go, and then came a chain reaction. What a thrill! We weren't going back to class. Furthermore, we would go room by room to liberate the whole school.

The look on the teachers' startled faces was beyond compare as a classroom's worth of us stormed the doorways and pre-empted the subject matter. Most of the hunched students were so doused in boredom that they needed shock treatment to sit up straight, and we delivered. "Strike! Strike! Strike!" we chanted, the syllable like a drumbeat calling. "Join us! Come on!"

In each room a brave few defied the rigid air of disapproval to stand up and come with us. Soon we were a small but mighty snake weaving down halls and chanting, "One, two, three, four, we don't want your fucking war!"

An adult from the office approached us and a dialogue began. Eventually the administration picked off the stragglers, and then their friends; soon almost everyone had been coaxed back to class. I knew I'd look the fool if I stood alone—or worse. Punishment would be swift for a lone troublemaker, a misfit, *a girl with mental problems.* Is that how they saw me? How much about my past did they know? I thought about what Barry said, and chided myself for nurturing individualized paranoia while in Southeast Asia the body count climbed.

As if my father were there to defend me, I came through it unscathed. Maybe I blended with the other loudmouths or maybe, for once, it wasn't about me; maybe, this being the San Francisco Bay area and all, there was sympathy among the teachers and they held the administration in check. Or maybe they knew I was a married student—a strange odd duck, yet untouchable. What if they knew about the B-Brothers and their activism? It would be like Osage End all over again—off the hook via connection to protective male power.

Privately, I had to laugh. The San Jose Liberation Front was nothing more than a dozen college-age idealists, at most. And Chris (my husband in name only) was no patriarch with any punch. He tried his best to lord it over me but came off like a puffy little rooster, pesky and shrill. That evening, when I admitted to the B-Brothers that well, er, we sort of went back to class and that was the end of it, there was more contempt for my husband than for sweet-sixteen.

Shortly after my stint as a strike-instigator we moved again, and I was left to come up with a diploma on my own. Chris had a falling out with Barry that affected the entire roommate dynamic, and we found ourselves in a tattered old neighborhood at the edge of downtown. I accepted the loss of my real revolutionaries with the same simmering fatalism that most of Chris' antics spawned, a sullen girl waiting for her chance to give surrogate-dad the slip.

While I would never be in Boogie's league, and while Brett stayed neutral, Barry's scorn for Chris was tough to behold. I felt contaminated by his judgment and accepted it as another stain spilled onto my soul, already bulging with self-disgust.

Faces I could not be

The new neighborhood was tense. Our building leaked in the rain. The only heat was from a small electric space heater. The family that lived below, junkies in recovery, tried to parent a son between screaming fits and tinkering with their methadone dosage. With my husband toiling at his job-of-the-month, I had time on my hands after following up on employment want ads myself. Unfortunately, it was only a short stroll to the radical bookstores, a direction I veered too often when I should have been looking for work.

There, on cheap newsprint, was more emotion than the big publishers could stand. Racks of black-and-white type set by local hands promised to give voice to people like me, or at least the person I wanted to be. In that bookstore I studied more than merchandise, stealing looks at women in berets, long-locked leaders, and a college kid wearing a vest of political buttons that sang a warrior's song. The uproar of local dissent spilled into those self-owned and operated publications, vibrant with fresh art and financed by storefront merchants from those very streets. I bought all kinds, feeling a mixture of guilt and titillation. I should have been reading classics like Marx and Mao, but wanted instead to crawl inside the passionate mind of the woman or man standing next to me.

One late afternoon the place was packed—my best opportunity for rubbing shoulders with the crowd. Students were down from the ivory tower and the street people had just awakened. A newspaper called *The Madness Network News* struck my eye. It displayed the characteristic ragged graphics and blotchy ink job, plus the tag line "All the fits that's news to print." I bought it without perusal, knowing full well that the B-Brothers would not approve. As much as I tried to expunge her, the ghost of Agnes still kept popping up, urging me to figure out my family disease once and for all.

Brett and Barry would never believe "mental health" to be more than a bourgeois concern. Their hero, Karl Marx, was fairly silent about the inner life; in his day asylums claimed the poor and, as Freud emerged into view, emotions were for the privileged few to contemplate. The only contemporary take on the subject to which the B-Brothers gave their stamp of approval was *One Flew over the Cuckoo's*

Nest, Ken Kesey's novel about the psychiatric institution as totalitarian regime. Barry, Brett, and even Boogie would surely counsel the psychiatrically oppressed to organize around the primary issue (smashing the state) and not simply psychiatry, one little finger of its grabbing hand. They would find the voices in *The Madness Network News* well intentioned, but too focused on lesser targets. Most often those targets were the purveyors of electroconvulsive therapy or, as Ernest Hemmingway put it after being forced into the treatment, *shock docs.*

I always wondered how Agnes Wohler Elton stood it: whether she asked for it (*punish me, punish me now*), whether they tricked her or reasoned with her, or baldly told her to lie down and get strapped in for the ride of her life. How could anyone misunderstand my grandmother so thoroughly, how could they refuse to sit with her and just listen? Zapping sweet old ladies with mega-volts of current to the brain had one purpose only: to obliterate thought of any kind. Forgetfulness as therapy. At what price? *The Madness Network News* thought it far too great.

Shock was like napalm, made to hurt, to teach a brutal lesson under the guise of greater good. It struck me that Ultra-revolutionary Barry was missing the parallel: if Vietnam dodged deadly flash-fire for "freedom," then shock treatment was the napalm of "mental health."

Photos in *The Madness Network News* showed the faces of the ex-inmates of psychiatry, those who'd learn to fight rather than to give up on dead-end wards. I cheered their tactics and verve, but something about their worn faces gave pause. I'd seen that look somewhere before.

That strange kid at the Habitat. And also on my brother Sam.

Maybe my mother was right: the move to Kansas had been disastrous for my big brother. We all dismissed the night-time screaming, the isolation from his peers, the long hours he spent laying on his bed, toes pointed to the ceiling as his feet traced the air back and forth. We dismissed it because Sam was the Brain. He did well at the lab school, that wing of the university where future teachers apprenticed, and our father assured us that brains meant that, in the end, you came out on top.

Although Chris and I skirted poverty, we always had our minds, our theories, and our membership in *the vanguard*. The City was full of our kind, the privileged poor. So I read on, protected, immune…and yet uneasy.

I read about protests at the offices of shock doctors. One of the latter maintained business-as-usual not far from the small radius where San Jose's head shops, radical bookstores, and second-hand clothing shops commingled. The shock doc's parking lot was hit hard by a steady gaggle of the formerly fried and drugged psychiatric survivors. This I had to see.

Curious but scared, I told myself I'd just pass by. My legs were strong and used to walking. I didn't even have to look, but I knew I would, if only from the corners of my eyes.

In minutes the doctor's parking lot gave itself away: there were the demonstrators, ten or so, carrying signs about the crimes of the man hiding inside. Something drew me closer as I looked for a place to hide and observe.

A leaflet-laden demonstrator caught my eye. "Here's the low-down on Doctor Shock," he said, thrusting the half-sheet at me. "How did you find out about us?"

It was too direct. A prod to join them would come next. Normally, I didn't miss a beat in grabbing up a sign. But something was wrong.

"Oh, I, uh…here," I said, holding up my just-purchased *Madness Network News*. "Bought it today—a good read!" I chirped, bright and false.

The leaflet man was honored. "Why, thank you," he blushed. "I write the San Jose coverage." But I was already head-down into the leaflet as if it were a map to buried treasure, which gave me time to step back to a retaining wall where onlookers sat with Marlboros and potato chips. I could overhear their conversation just above me.

"Why do they ever let these people out of the hospital?"

"Because they lie. Play the game. Take their meds into zombie-land, then chuck 'em in the garbage when sprung at last."

"The doc needs a drive-through window right over there. You should be so lucky to operate it. When's your last day at State anyway?"

The leaflet blurred before my eyes as I realized that these were Doctor Shock's employees on break, enjoying the show. Maybe they had just attended a jolting inside—or did they only do that at the hospitals? I deliberately turned my entire body away from them, still feigning absorption in the text of the leaflet. It was a maddening impasse.

The demonstrators were my watershed moment of truth. If I stood with them, then the Wohler Madness was oppression; Agnes could be vindicated. Yet what did that make me, the Habitat graduate who'd moved on to a more sweeping analysis of the culture's woes? What did it make Sam, who I knew was a brain but not right in the head?

And how could Sam's fate be my father's fault? The two of them never fought, unlike the two of us. Sam had unceasingly approved of my father, who, although he didn't quite know what to make of his son's *introspective* behavior, encountered no guff there. Our parents came off as overprotective for letting Sam be Sam—friendless, pissed, perpetually *in potential*. I thought of Boogie's rapture over R.D. Laing. I'd never noticed Sam's scientific mind pushing for some inner journey that anyone ever tried to squelch. So what were the politics of the Wohler Madness experience? Where was the visionary in our bloodline, and who was to blame for taking him down?

The pressure to sort it out was too great. These people had suffered—and probably not on daddy's insurance money. They'd been through the worst of every treatment medical psychiatry concocted and had lived to tell about it—they *had* to tell about it, or perhaps go mad for good. They were not my tribe of rebellious, pot-smoking kids who hated their parents. We weren't worthy to touch their signs. In them I recognized the true suffering I'd seen in my grandmother and brother, even though I'd tried to explain both as casualties of capitalism.

Where did I fit? I wanted to stand with them, support them, weep for them, and rejoice at the same time, yet I stayed frozen to the concrete wall. Much as I wanted to embrace mad pride, I didn't want it to embrace me. I pored over the printed words because I could not look directly at the brave and the broken. I escaped the Wohler Madness without a telltale mark, with no overdose of sadistic electrical current that might change my thinking about humanity forever. I was a foot-loose revolutionary who could choose any cause that inspired me. I had paid few dues.

And yet there *was* a netherworld that claimed me. I wasn't like the B-Brothers or their girlfriends, and hardly like the bored kids in my California high school, ripe for the picking to *strike!* Because Agnes was institutionalized, and the legacy of the famous Wohler veered beyond his scientific accomplishments, I was marked. I hated Doctor Shock's henchmen laughing above the scene, but at least I could walk away. For now.

So I did.

"Thanks for stopping by!" the leaflet man yelled. As I spun around, he looked into my soul. I raised a clenched fist in solidarity and several demonstrators responded in kind. It made me feel better.

But it wasn't enough.

PART TWO
LUNAR SANE

Chapter 5
MOON OVER FLINT

It wasn't an easy climb, grabbing twine over needle-sharp grass. The cylinders of prairie hay were rolled to eye level, but wider than my arms could stretch. I could have plunked into a lawn chair, but sitting atop these bales was the best place to watch the night.

In darkness the Flint Hills of Kansas are bare bumps cut through by shallow streams, willows and cottonwoods erasing private properties. My only neighbor was beyond the skinny and scant Verdigris River, then down a slope. No light or sound from their place made it through the night as the moon rose over crabapple branches in the yard.

This beat sitting in a quiet house. A house emptied of marriage: my second try, on a farmstead that an Osage End native and I had rented with such high hopes. We fell apart before the barn heard more than the crowing of two roosters without a harem. During our last pointless fight I ordered my spouse to get out, and he complied. Each day since I'd tried to take it back. Twice divorced before the age of thirty! I was beginning to feel like a stereotype, summed up in the prairie vernacular: *rode hard and put away wet.*

This time was different than my uncoupling from Chris Glen. That failed revolutionary and I became our own version of Tricky Dick and the Vietnamese. While Chris teetotaled and bragged about it— not out of a well-versed platform of sobriety, but because it made him different from everyone else with long hair—I inhaled and ingested and took lovers on the sly. Spouse became parental watchdog, and I retaliated with a practiced form of guerilla warfare that drew upon my Habitat tricks.

Chris' constant warnings about my inability to live alone rang false with me at last. Apolitical and aimless, my husband lost every job and every place to live that he took a notion to procure for us. At least he had a mission: to keep tabs on me. At the age of nineteen I ended it, and tried to take on San Francisco on my own.

The City was loud and crazy, packed with possibilities. Simply looking at the Sunday paper brought on an anxiety attack—so many fascinating events, how to choose? I pumped gas for a living and slept with a customer or two, but knew this place could never be home. In time the loneliness became excruciating. I considered it no defeat to head back to the front porch of the Flint Hills.

Without Chris to battle, I was stuck with no gumption and no plan. My father asked me to come home after I spilled the beans about the wasteland inside. In a massive and sudden reversal, nostalgia for my prairie roots rushed into the void.

But during countless nights atop that scratchy hale bale, I missed husband number two. He'd been the real reason for my return. We had courted through letters between California and Kansas, and he was such an improvement over Chris Glen—or so I thought. Until I realized I had traded in the Controller for the Confirmed Loner. A loner with a penchant for cruising in his truck, asking women on the street if they'd like a ride.

After I threw him out there was no more drama to distract me, and things went downhill. It had been years since I'd taken the Wohler Madness seriously and a decade since I'd lived in the Elton house. One divorce, especially in California, was a badge of experience, but a repeat this soon meant nothing less than failure. I moped and wondered if the family disease was sneaking in the back door. Sleep was becoming a habit again, and killer migraines knocked me out twice a month. But unlike with Agnes, there was no one to take me to the hospital. And unlike Agnes, I'd rather die than go there. What next?

California dreamin' intensified as I scrunched down into the hay and wondered if Chris was right. Had I really failed by returning here? Once back in Kansas, I had no idea what to do with the future besides pursuing romance, but there was always that troubling need to pay the rent. I knew how to take refuge in school and had a flair for obtaining loans—I was the professional student whose need to tarry flatters but unsettles the tenured staff. What a way to put off the proving ground and still pass for promising.

The odd jobs that supported this limbo were the famous time-wasters of life. That night I had returned from the latest in a series of hateful endeavors, yet another mind-numbing stint waiting tables where the fare was Midwest steak and potatoes attended by hopelessly over-boiled corn.

It was so difficult to mingle day after day with the average bears.

Osage End was the same as when I left it. The university where my father taught still exercised limited influence on the town's demeanor. Sprawling factories drew people in with hefty wages and then shoved them out with chronic pain and mood swings. Aside from dodging that fate, what kept me hanging in with school?

Oh, that's right: I wanted to become a teacher. The crabapple doesn't fall very far from the tree. But what public school would have me instruct their kids? Or more to the point, which dull building in which dull little town could I stand to be in for more than a day?

I should have been working on a resume instead of lolling on hay, waiting for the moon. Still, this was far less humiliating than my other pastime: driving by my spouse's apartment, imagining him inside, revving the engine up and down the block. Pissed off as hell. How could he leave me alone with myself this way?

But it was autumn now in the limestone hills, there was a fine moon, and all of that could wait. In the fields of tenant farmers, summer gave up the ghost. Stubble pointed at angles, blackening, the expanse wide and stark and bruised from agri-machines. Over this bleak slate the moon rose perfectly round, orange on its first steps up.

The contrast between this landscape and beaches backed by mountains still came to mind. But the pang was growing softer. I knew this moon; the one in California belonged to someone else. This moon was mine from the first time cousins and I saddled our horses at midnight on our grandparents' farm. When the land and I got together, concepts like failure and defeat were forced to keep their distance.

A few miles away, in Osage End, my brothers still orbited the Elton home. Ben was a motor-head teenager. Sam had graduated with a degree in physics and stepped into the work world. He was a researcher at some industry in Kansas City, testing products, quality control, something I didn't understand. As when we were little, he couldn't fully explain it to my untutored mind.

Big brother always seemed angry, stoppered, ready to blow. He was perpetually overweight but loomed even larger, a fortress barricaded by the familiar Elton contempt, still with that unnerving habit of constantly jiggling one leg up and down. But that was just Sam, we pretended. So the shock was total when he took his first real dive off the deep end. One that left no room for excuses anymore, one that set his course forever. I couldn't push the scenario out of my mind yet, even in the dark hills, safe and alone.

The mantle is passed

I'd been hired to do lawn care for a church when one day my father pulled into its deserted weekday lot. Robert Elton and I were pals now, ever since my return from California. It was a truce called with cordiality—plus an implied pact to never discuss the past. In the hot Indian summer my father walked over with his head nearly bowed. A reticent gait, shoulders at half-mast—it was ominous. None of the usual swagger that conveyed, *Oh there you are, cutting grass and almost a college graduate…when **are** you going to graduate?*

I did a quick search of possibilities. My dad was fairly blasé about the second divorce. Neither of my husbands had played the son-in-law who adored him. Nor would he slowly trudge the gravel parking lot in the event of a death or accident. I figured there was no emergency—his pace was downright labored. In fact, he looked beaten.

At least the heart attacks were behind him. Triple bypass surgery, and he'd slid by the reaper. He walked a mile a day and lived what is called a normal life, if somewhat solitary and routine.

Veering from his usual trajectory—school to home, and back again—violated the rhythm of things. Had I done something horribly wrong? No, those weren't clouds of rage gathering about the now-thinning hair, the bald spot combed across with a few strands. My father stood before his daughter, who held a cheap electric weedwhacker in front of a—gasp—Protestant church.

"It's Samuel," he said.

"What happened?"

"He quit his job, drove that Chevy Vega all the way to Portland, Oregon. Tried to board a ship to leave the country."

How hard to name the thickness, the stickiness of the silence that follows that kind of news. Brothers who were smarter than the above-average bear and worked for corporations didn't do the inexplicable.

"But—why on earth?"

"He thought his boss was plotting to kill him."

I unplugged the machine and regarded the length of orange cord. Then I stared at my dad.

He wanted something from me, something he should have gotten from someone else. He wanted me to feel sorry for him, absolve him, share his burden, take some shape of the sorrow away.

"And his boss, surely not…"

"Oh jeez, no. Sam was just a small cog in the giant wheels of that place; his boss barely knew he existed. He just—Sam's just…"

There were those beseeching eyes again. I felt a weight on my chest. The family disease. It had a name but we never spoke it, not like the other one that shaped the family discourse: *heart attack, triglycerides, lipid profiles, oh my!* We left it to psychiatrists to name the flavors of our disgrace: depression, paranoia, mania, doomed. It was odd—my father always filled the air space, usually with assured pronouncements about how things work or why a favored plan will work. Then I got it: suddenly it was my job. My head reeled with the responsibility, and the audacity. After years of corking it, was I required to speak on this subject?

Robert Elton was not going to finish his sentence; he wanted me to do it. Maybe the Habitat gave me status as a guest expert? Maybe my utterance of some clinical phrase, or even the words "mentally ill," meant that I had accepted our inevitable scourge. I understood and it was okay that, once upon a time, they thought I was the one who had it bad, that I was Wohler-mad.

Mute as a stone I stood my ground, on someone else's dandelion and fescue. Habitat scenes flew by my inner eye. How they urged us to talk, talk, talk in group therapy, but when we did—nothing but ridicule, scorn, censure. Dismissed. Now I was either going to speak with that voice, or use that of the Helpers. Neither one would work, nor could I pull off the dutiful daughter: Aw, there, there, daddykins, how sad you are!

So, one question. The only question.

"What are you going to do?"

It was the query of an outsider. Despite an apparent invitation, I would never really be part of the family again, not after Denver, the Habitat, California, and the marriages that failed. I didn't dream of asking, *what are we going to do?* Quick to remove Agnes and me to a place for fixing, they merely waited while their number-one son shrank further and further from his own life. Until Sam figured it out: You can't hide, but you can run.

From the few bits of news that fell into my ears during the California hiatus, I could see this coming. Without university life, Sam's social isolation had deepened considerably. But Robert and Marie Elton could not admit that their son's growing paranoid behavior warranted concern. Now, what they would do was already decided. I'd neither co-conspire nor comment.

"Get him some help, I guess," sighed my father, turning up his palms at his sides for one dogged second. "There's a hospital in Kansas City…"

A familiar crossroads: the descent of the family disease. It had to pick someone. Agnes was an elderly fixture in a nursing home, contained and no threat. Sue was going to school and working for a wage. While my father described the extent of Sam's agitation, I put the weed-whacker down and crossed my arms, my eyes racing over the cracks in the pavement because I couldn't meet the ones upon me. Had I looked at my father, I would have seen it: *You're excused. It's not you. Not anymore.* Thus the heir to the Wohler Madness moved up to take his place in line; Agnes was finished, and someone needed to do it. How close I had come to being the one.

Words were not pearls I could string together right then, so I settled for the frozen face of surprise that this could be happening to Sam.

I felt my father deflate even further because I didn't soothe his pain or try to sop it up with female concern. How could I? With the new truce we were equals, I thought. I met him halfway by being like him, but I wouldn't take on what felt like the subservient role of confidant about a matter we had never addressed together: me and the mental hospital. Yet although I didn't show it, it was there: pity for my father's loneliness. Sure, I felt like a heel. But the urge to hold back was stronger, *after all he did to me.*

Robert Elton turned and walked over to his immaculate car, glancing back with a half-smile and a wave to acknowledge that it was okay. At least I'd done something—I'd listened. Sort of. He could always pretend.

Ultimate Dad above

The fact of Sam's illness made anguishing over a second divorce seem a bit overwrought. My brother was running from a murderer who didn't exist, while I simply couldn't keep a man. I knew my heartbreak wasn't the Wohler Madness—I didn't hear voices, I thought melodramatically about suicide but wouldn't dare (the hazy Thorazine episode of the Habitat aside, a lark gone wrong). So it never occurred to me to call it crazy, delusional, or schizoid when everything changed at the edge of a fallow field that night. What happened with the moon over a swath of Flint Hills completely bypassed the Wohler Madness. It set up a whole new ballpark a million miles from that old duality: crazy or sane?

Because it went against everything the rationalist in me stood for. Despite doing our Catholic duty on Sunday, there was nothing spiritual about growing up in the Elton home. Spiritual wasn't smart.

Besides, finding out you could not literally see God in church was a disappointment I never recovered from. It happened one Sunday on the way home from mass, during our Mur's book-throwing days in Kentucky. "God wore green today," I remarked from the back seat. The laughter in the car was howling, but good-natured; I'd thought the priest was Him! But it was just a man up there in a shiny robe. Billowing and decorated, but just a man.

Once I heard that the real deal was invisible, had superpowers, and was always watching *me*, how could the child not wait, poised for God the Father to do the same thing as fathers of daughters. Exalt the bond, but so easily get pissed off? Punish capriciously? Demand to be number one and scorn all competitors?

And so it was that in Osage End, Kansas, not long after coveting the faces on my mother's ladies' magazine, the shortcomings of God the Father put the Catholic Church on my list of totally irrelevant stuff. There was a parallel between Daddy here and Daddy Above Unseen.

I didn't like what He supposedly asked of his supposed only son, and I didn't believe that son willingly went along. Fear incubated in me over the Jesus story as I sat beneath the thorn-studded, crucified, nearly naked man with dripping blood and tortured face. It was a lot like television, the death and the gore. During the boring parts of mass I thumbed through the missal and read about the martyrs. Same story, time and again. Somebody got hurt or killed, all glory to God. That was supposed to make me feel loved?

When I was fifteen, I'd had enough. I woke up one morning acknowledging what had been building for months: I had no belief in God. It was a move that felt way smarter than the average bear. Time to inform my family that, as an atheist, I would no longer attend church.

I waited until a Sunday morning. Adjusting my flannel nightgown to its full queenly length, I assumed an advantage as I lurked in bed, inviolable under piles of blankets. But I was wrong. My mother knocked for the usual wake-up call. I delivered my edict and she stared. Then turned and shut the door.

One minute. Two. You know footsteps are angry by the way they nick the stairs, like Harvard Classics hitting the floor. A sound doubly strange because this parent never came up to our rooms. The house was old and the stairwell narrow. It was navigable, but claustrophobic. When I heard my father hit the postage-stamp landing, I practiced my speech again. Surely, as a fighter and a rationalist, he would see the reason behind this. So I started talking first.

"How can there be a God or heaven? I'm not going inside a church again. Not today, or ever. It doesn't make sense! I don't feel anything—and neither do you."

That may have been going too far. What did I expect to come next, a thoughtful discussion of theology? But the deist who slid into

Catholicism only to appease the future in-laws took the whole thing viscerally.

I watched my father flush red, a Class-A rage at hand. His wordless rebuke was more like a snarl: a hand on my wrist yanking me out of bed, my shoulder hitting the nearby wall—it all took less than five seconds. We would not be late for church. I simmered and found suitable clothes, carrying my hatred inside the sanctuary like contraband, a stash that I would someday make good on.

After I married Chris Glen, I was never asked to go to mass again. This was fortunate, since I believed revolutionaries should be consumed with more important thoughts than religion. Being seen in church bucked the rebel-girl image of myself that I clung to like a life raft. The good fight was my anchor, the devil a phony opponent. There were plenty for real in the Blah World that needed standing up to.

Soon enough after coming back to Kansas, I found an opponent—a pair of utilities bent on building a fission reactor too close for comfort. Farmers and city environmentalists protested the nuclear plant slated for cornfields a few short miles from Osage End. The specter of the nuke was immediate, and I embraced the chance to do something concrete with people from all walks of life. But in the end they built the thing and fired it up. The vanguard dispersed, all at loose ends.

What next?

The shine that spoke

Is that why I commenced talking to the moon as if it were a sentient, breathing, listening body? As if it was the face of something all-seeing and wise?

There would always be the next struggle for justice. The vanguard would reconfigure. But was I going to go through those motions again? Too many endings: California, divorce, the latest tribe lost. I just wanted to sit outside and do…nothing. But something outside had other ideas. I sensed an invitation.

Say I came to the moon because I had to slog through the mire first. Say I was out of options. Just don't say I was grasping at straws. Because, while I always fancied the fringe elements, I never hoped to fall so far as religion. Spirituality? Was that just a different word that permitted wider interpretations? Or had environmentalism developed a devotional side and I was infected with its possibilities?

I looked at the moon from the top of that cylinder of hay, and to that looming face I laid it all out: every nook of pain, how high the stakes, how certain the dead end. I talked to the moon like it was my confessor, but I was in no mind to do penance. I poured forth the bulk of sorrowful shame that was crowding me and sent it through miles of empty space. Driven, risking, pleading—I spread the air with grief and dread. But with a twist, trying on another uncomfortable word: faith. Faith that something vast was out there, able to turn the tide.

In my mind a sneaky taunt began: *what desperation will drive a gal to do.* But that niggling cynic forever shut her trap when the moon answered back.

It was only the moon, hanging there the same as ever, but the very tone of the reply shattered me. I didn't have to squint or blink to know I wasn't seeing things, because the moon shone unchanged. No lips formed on its surface, no crater fixed me with a terrible eye, no blaze of light filled the sky. Just a voice.

It was outside, and seemed to come from the moon. It was inside, and seemed to come from the moon.

You are neither insane nor about to kill yourself. Come back to me, She said.

The voice was female.

She!?! Shapes in the night clicked into silver clarity. I was too seized by the moment to question the voice or the gender donned by the Moon—I was Saul struck down on the road to Damascus by a sweet face in the sky, given no mission but to stop bashing my own mind. By God, it was She! I couldn't sort out which fact astounded me more: not only was something out-there/in-here, reassuring and revelatory, and not only was the One speaking to me, but it was female!

To be so suddenly seen *and* to have my marital woes so thoroughly preempted, to feel blissfully singled out as the only woman on a hay bale on this night, by these fields, yet somehow profoundly aware of a self erased, ended and yet starting anew. I turned the nougat of gold over and over in my mind. It was simply and clearly knowing this: that I was as much part and parcel of every element of nature I could see, smell, hear, and sense in the dark.

Thus spake the Moon.

I slid off the hay bale and tried to decide—was I nuts? But the moon's presence wasn't fleeting. I knew what crazy was—anything but bliss. We did it with anguish and inertia in our family, and I was miles from either. So I spent until midnight just basking, walking the harvest ruts and explaining, curling up and giving the soil some hearty shouts and some tears. Letting it all go. Being held in Her shine and hearing that life was never going to be the same.

In torn topsoil that harbored stalk and pesticide, I found out where I was supposed to be. *Here.* I was supposed to be here. I wasn't soiling the planet, ruining minds, ruining myself, wasting potential, or hurting anyone in particular. I wasn't poison. I was here.

I still expected an entrance from the cynical viper I knew so well, that scoffer from my own mind who would crate the whole thing away, sneering wide. But the critic was stumped. The moment stayed blessedly safe from analysis.

The freedom, for once, not to require experience to undergo a strip-search in front of the guards of rationality. The relief of knowing that we are not Existential Man, all losers, scooting about trying to get more money, more stuff, more sex, then going dead as a doornail. The permission to be other than my father's daughter, but knowing that this transcended rebellion against him. Crazy? This madness was divine. I wasn't being told I was Jesus, or to kill anyone, or that the government was tapping my phone. That was the best thing She said: *This is no Wohler Madness. Welcome home to your right mind.*

Who She was

When I finally slipped into bed, smiling for the first time since the spouse had cleared out, I did what any Elton would do: I decided to get some references. By now the moon was on "her" way to the other side of the world, and dawn would break soon. Bolting up and forsaking a good sleep, I pillaged for a book I'd carted along through move after move, a gift from some boyfriend between marriages. I never cracked it because it seemed…too weird? Too esoteric? It was a book about the moon.

Moon, Moon by Anne Kent Rush is a rush for the senses, a book that skips over coffee-table pretense and goes for the heart of art. The author loved the Moon more than I ever knew I could, and went looking for all things lunar in countless cultures. She found The Goddess. This was more than I'd bargained for. But the voice had to be Someone. I couldn't call Her "God" without wincing.

In the weeks that followed, between waitressing, yard work, and night dreams of Goddess temples, I sank into that book, went up onto the hay bale—-and kept talking to the moon. Waiting for the upshot, waiting to start acting really stupid, megalomaniacal. Or schizophrenic. Waiting to hear, *They're out to get you! They have your phone tapped! They will kill you!* Then it would really be true: whack job, the Wohler Madness.

Instead, I slowly put myself together. I leaned on more than the Moon—I thanked all that was around me, these old Flint Hills and their ways. Or maybe the Moon directed me to regard Her treasures anew, the landscape She watched over by night and halftime, day.

I couldn't separate the sky and land as this phrase kept swirling into my thoughts: Goddess as prairie.

Here were the worn low hills and their wild occupants as I'd never seen them before. Husband number two was an artist; though he claimed our marriage halted his craft, he had taught me a thing or two about Kansas. Dutifully I had tried to look with his eyes from pastures to photographs to sketches and back again—but I still longed for sand and madrone. With the lunar face over Flint to guide me, I got it: all of Her body is beautiful.

The soft speak of tall grass in a wind, the subtlety of its rust tones. The deer ambling up to the edge of the yard, standing and looking. The great blue heron at the pond that let me come close. The Moon said, *See the quail flying toward you in the river's small woods, listen to the scratch of mice in your walls. We know Each Other.* I learned to drop the story that I was monumentally alone with my own mind and precious self-pity. I listened to what the whole world was saying and singing.

And from a cache of books that make it into very few history classrooms, The Goddess emerged. Life-giver, holy pregnant Mother, rainmaker and crop-giver, moon moon. What She meant to people was unmistakably more compassionate than the Yahweh story. She meant for them to dance, love, make stories, grow, and get stoned on Her beauty. Was it such a coincidence that there was a match in antiquity between Her worship and the high status of women?

Could you really do religion this way? No "true believer" status required, no lock-step ritual scripts, no assigned peer group, no rules to stay inside a building in order for the spirit to fly? I could trust Her, for she was not just a man conducting church in a silken green dress.

This changes everything

Agitating in the streets, in boardrooms and bedrooms for women's rights was one thing. As if women had no history before the suffrage push, but knew they could make a future. They were knocking on a door and asking for a chance to prove themselves.

But it took courage to dig and deliver a most astounding history/herstory out of the archaic past, and I was grateful to those who made the leap. To grasp that, for most of humanity's lifespan in diverse places, God was a woman and women the natural leaders? It changed the way I looked at men.

Some feared that modern Goddess women wished to do away with the patriarchy but keep the same rules of domination, substituting a change of personnel to make a *matriarchy*. Inside the heart of the Goddess, where lying on Her earth formed my nights after days spent looking into Her past, the thought was laughable. What had Goddess women ever done to men by force? Men were the force experts, the war, rape, and poverty experts. Which of these power-over ploys could be laid at any matriarchy's door?

What astonished me was the role for men that emerged under the primacy of the moon and all She stood for. Lovers, brothers, and sons all on board with this. Frankly, it was beyond the modern woman's grasp. The immersion in art, ceremony, children, play, craft, earth and sky wasn't divvied up into separate belongings, his versus hers. Another striking feature of this hidden past: the further one went back in time, the more one noted the lack of weapons, warfare, and fortifications against enemies. It gave new meaning to the phrase "paradise lost." What if paradise was once a place and people as real as these Flints and its inhabitants?

This changed everything. I stopped driving by the ex's house so much. I went to see my parents more, and quit interrupting my father to interject my own views. There was less of a need to trawl for male approval at every turn.

But it wasn't easy to talk about my real and pressing dialogues with what most people classed as mere scenery. My priorities were not on human discourse—and what a needed break that was. I was being spoken to by wind, sun, rain, and wildlife.

The prairie. The Moon.

To meet Her own

The need for tribe was bound to re-surface. Chris Glen had soured me on the rhetoric of revolution, and where was the "Left" in the Flint Hills of Kansas anyway? I was more interested in locating women like the writer who'd birthed *Moon, Moon*. Where did they live, how did they carry on with one another? I couldn't imagine a thing such as—cringe—"worship," fearing it would be like church with the Divine Mother in place of Sky Pops. Another fake party speaking in Goddess tongues under the full moon.

But what if these women were onto something else? Something older, something recovered, something of the wild mystic's way before the advent of cathedral and pew?

At first I found a way to eavesdrop: periodicals. In their pages I was intrigued to find even tougher words than Goddess: *Pagan, witch*.

Into my mailbox came the modern-day Pagans. I couldn't relate to a lot of it. It seemed like fairytale fantasizing, and I was still a hard-nosed politico under it all. But when they weren't calling attention to themselves or praising their own "magical skills," the Pagans' sentiment toward the earth as Goddess seemed sincere. I wondered even more just who these people might be in real life. I vowed to meet them.

I worried, however, about pursuing this line of thought as a resident of the Bible Belt. I never actually saw the mail carrier that traversed the county in a cloud of dust; the house sat a long lane's curve away from my mailbox. Discreet brown wrappers cloaked the Pagan periodicals, but when people populate sparsely, they can be nosy. Among the chemically enhanced farms, the Saturday pheasant hunters and Sunday holy-rollers, my tie with the college wasn't much cover. I happened to know how they felt about Satan in these parts: he was alive and well in anyone who missed church.

But I was so far removed from the fabric of rural community my house might have been a monastery. With so little to lose, I thought I'd go for broke and meet some of these Pagans.

Just to see if I was turning into someone who might leave Kansas again.

Or figure out how to live here while She turned on the lights in my brain and soothed some scars on the heart.

Chapter 6
DIVINE MADNESS

Three witches chanting in the rental car and me—sick, so sick. Oncoming headlights doing needlepoint along my eyebrows, a migraine's vascular squeeze. Nausea that should be cradled in bed, in a dark room, not a minivan filled with song, curving and swerving along California's coastal Highway One.

This was the only way to reach Cedar Wing, the woman who named herself after a tree and a bird. Write a book and they will come: her event was held at a rambling farmhouse rented to forty registrants, most of us pitching tents in the pines. But first came the arduous trip, switching planes, meeting a carpool headed by an imperious crone rumored to be independently wealthy. Then it was dark, with torrents of rain along the coast, and I didn't know any of the words to the songs.

The women tried to give me aspirin, useless at that point. I was a statue at my window, praying through each blind curve for my guts to hold on one minute longer. Suddenly, the Goddess gave me a break.

On a turnout across the road, a young man struggled with a motorcycle that had fallen in the muck. My witches were energized and eager to show good will. They pulled over and ran to help the startled rider on his way, while I made a beeline for the edge of the road and puked to the whitecaps below.

At last we pulled up to Juggernaut Farm. A contingent came out to greet us, pulled by an obvious leader. She approached our driver, the mouthy elder, with kisses and hugs. The rest of us were summarily squeezed and told, "The ritual is about to begin."

There'd been no picture on the book jacket, so I asked She Who Spoke for All, "Who are you?"

"Cedar Wing," she answered, with only a dash of irritation that added: *And you should have known that.*

Inside the farmhouse, hardwood floors stretched across a living room free of clutter and furnishings. We lowered ourselves onto that floor and out of the mundane. With Cedar Wing in charge, magic was never made on sofas and chairs. Our carpool completed the assembly, which now formed a perfectly circular shape. I noticed men present, a small minority looking pleased and at ease. Everyone made room as we hunkered down and our leader began.

"We'll go around the circle and each one of us will sing our name. Then we'll sing it back to you."

Migraine made way for pure terror. But somehow I got through it, soft breathy syllables straining for more lilt than croak. When I said I was from Kansas, everybody laughed.

Between each vocal spotlight I made a covert study of Cedar Wing. She'd described herself as part Native American—from her looks, it was hard to tell which part. Flaming red hair, eyes of blue, and the palest skin to match made it easier to see her Celtic side. Yet she shone in her turquoise and silver, big cuffs of it at wrists and throat that she wore with a sense of entitlement. Not to mention the earrings.

Many of the other women had them, too—long, dangly, substantial, and entirely beaded earrings. No two designs alike, none available in any store. Each day of Pagan Boot Camp, Cedar Wing wore the longest and most original design. Consequently her earlobes were pendulous, and but for the thick and curly hair it was hard not to stare.

Such thoughts were flicked aside by the call to action. We hung on every word as Cedar Wing spoke.

"These are weeks of power for our selves. Women hide their spirits while taking care of the world, their families, and everybody else. Men do it, too. I hope you've left Little Mister and Miss Doing-For behind—they're not good traveling companions for sliding between the worlds.

"What these workings can do, this magic, is bend and shape us. Take us into the raw clay of tomorrow, where you fashion your outcomes. Elements class, you're our babies. New to the dance, that's you—and we'll show you some various ways to step your beginnings. In fact, we'll do that right now in a ritual of welcoming. We're storming the heart of the Goddess with love. Her priestesses and priests have returned."

Whoops and hollering of joy, feet paddling the hardwood, silver jewelry flying everywhere. We all liked the sound of that.

Then the circle rose as one. Cedar Wing instructed us in taking root. She told how powerful the imagination was—that a woman or a man or any Witch could become, behind closed eyes, a tree. With sustained deep breathing we were led to feel the taproot or filigree spread, pushing down into soil from the soles of our feet. It would always be as a tree that we rooted—later, a sunny day on the land, we would plant real seedlings and trance into their fledgling pine leaves. But this tree was the Tree of Life.

I'm drawn to this stuff, I realized at that moment, *because I can't live in just one world.* The Tree was one of many things that ended up being Three.

Hanging out with witches and pagans, I was to learn the power of the number three. I recalled the veneration of the Holy Trinity from Catholic school—everybody knows something about a mighty three. Cedar Wing told us that Three reaches beyond the ping-pong of duality—this or that, black or white, young or old—to integration. The simple act of imagining oneself fully rooted and branched as a tree had all the symbolism a newbie could handle that night.

Roots stood for the unknown mystery-place, an initiation world that defies rational thought. The practical trunk meets everything above ground, the world where most live. Branches heave and sigh in a different spirit-realm—no more profound than darkness is the place saturated by light. Three worlds, none more esoteric or real-deal than the next. Then Cedar Wing told us to go full circuit: see what happens when the branches arc to touch the Earth.

And that was just the "grounding," to get us in the mood.

The ritual per se began with an open-eyed marking of territory. We faced east as one body, then south, west, and north. I thought I knew from Cedar Wing's books what meaning corresponded with each. That night, it was too much for me to keep straight: air/east/mind, fire/south/energy, water/west/emotion, earth/north/body, and then the Center where they mingle, where the ineffable lies, a cauldron of potential. Members of the Cadre (fellow teachers and witches from Cedar Wing's coven) blessed the space with incense, candle, water, and salt at each of the walls we were imagining so far beyond. When we faced the center again, it seemed like everyone but me called out a sacred name. "Isis, the healer…Cybele of the drum…Gaia Our Mother Earth…Freya, lover…Changing Woman…Hulda, Danu, Oya…" I shivered to hear praises so long forgotten now filling up the room.

Cedar Wing and the Cadre formed a gauntlet with arms raised like London Bridges, and we walked through singing, a winding snake of sorcerer's apprentices, whereupon we became circular again for the signature spiral dance. As the singing peaked and came to a satisfied halt, tired but happy, we passed a kiss with "Thou Art Goddess" all around. The Cadre showed us how to release the circle by thanking each of the elements and singing the sacred space goodbye for now.

With that, we were sent to our tents under one sliver of moon.

It was alternately safe and awkward to be one of the innocents at the practice of magic. At age 30, I was also one of the youngest there. Wide-eyed neophyte from Kansas was a hat I always wore well. When the witches took over Juggernaut Farm for two weeks, it was impossible to fake anything; no book learning could substitute for down-home ritual magic and oral transmission. You had to be there.

For starters, anyone could speak their mind and often did. Each morning we took to the hardwood floor for a "check in." On the second day Cedar Wing remarked, almost to herself, "No one's talking to me. It's like 'she's the one who wrote the book,' so they give a wide berth." From that moment on, something eased and released. I was impressed by how she did it, again and again, in little ways.

Like right after breakfast, tripping down the trail each day, I passed Cedar Wing who would announce, "Time for my morning shit!" Back then, she seemed a tad too proud of her regularity; now, I think she was just reminding us that she, too, darkened the outhouse door.

What also brought her "down" to our unpublished, untouted level was the Cadre. The other teachers had absolutely no truck with the Cedar Wing mystique. They were gladly in on the conspiracy to (playfully) knock her down a peg on occasion. They modeled respect balanced with camaraderie.

There was Maia, Cedar Wing's roommate back in the city, and her second in command. Maia was the flamboyant side of the more reserved "Cede," as she called her, when they worked in tandem. She made up for wearing petite size clothing with a booming voice that back home we'd call "husky." Maia talked about the book she would write as though she were every bit as good as her famous roomy. It was Maia who steered the babies, those total beginners in the Elements class. "I love to see people get this for the first time."

There was Athena, soon to dive into academe with her love for Russian literature; she was the overt lesbian, the cut-up, the vulnerable one. There was Griffin, a man with moon face and a fine guitar, loved (not at all secretly) by Maia. Ravenstar, the gay Jamaican cook, put raisins in every dish and taught us about herbs and oils on the side. And there was Bloudewedd.

Bloudewedd brought the only child into our midst, a three-year-old male son who clung to her nervously. It was clear that "B-wedd," as she was called, was not happy with the arrangement, although the rest of the camp did their best to take the pressure off mother by warming to the boy. The estranged papa had backed out of childcare at the last minute, and while B-wedd looked every bit the thin, blond image of the Celtic Flower Maiden, her sharp glances and wry one-liners only softened during actual "class" time.

One afternoon I excused myself from class with cramps, bad. In my tent, I awoke in fetal position to raised voices on the way to the privy. It was B-wedd and her son. Thinking all the campers engaged back at the farmhouse, she was in the midst of a tongue-lashing at high volume. It had a decidedly literary bent. There were many big words like "preposterous," which only fed the boy's wail and lament. Her fury and scorn paralyzed me inside the tiny pup tent, where I was dead sure I'd be charred next if I made a single sound.

Edgy, pissed, and driven, B-wedd was clearly on the fringes of the Cadre. Eventually, the storm brewing between her and Cedar Wing broke loose. By the end of camp she was history.

How do you become a pagan woman? Magic, magic, magic. Newly moonstruck in the Flint Hills of eastern Kansas, I read and read but never attempted a ritual. I would have felt so stupid. Always embarrassed in church when the faithful looked anything but reserved, my intellect was a jailer for spirituality's altered states. But at Pagan Boot Camp, everything went topsy-turvy for the poor ego. I learned that magic was always afoot alongside every mundane moment. I'd had an inkling of it among the Flint Hills when I was alone, sprung from the prison of rationalism, following deer tracks to the pond where heron fished the edge.

Among those forty witches and wannabes at the camp, there was a sense of imperative. Disenchantment with church-religion was one thing. But peeling back layers of myth and history to find one's home was another. Excavation, innovation.

For most of us, first steps began inside the covers of an orderly and finite book. Therein we found the bedrock for trust. Cedar Wing did two things with her seminal text, though at Boot Camp she neither pushed nor quoted the work. In its pages she railed at war, planet-destruction, and patriarchy, *and* she offered a mighty myth for setting things right.

The Goddess. Despite all the political and social potential in a female God, there was also the very personal homecoming to one's body. The images from archaic times ran the gamut in body types. Not only that, but they merged with animal, plant, or stylistic markings (such as for the life-giving rain) in a way that suggested the body was so much more than a separate object to sculpt and pluck at, a burden to carry through one's days.

Why did certain women see the possibilities in this, while others cringed? The occasional feminist aversion to Venus figures unearthed from Paleolithic and Neolithic times was based on an assessment of those icons as the sexual fantasies of cavemen. But why must you project a Playboy mentality back to the beginning of time, asked modern-day priestesses, when it's well documented that early humans thought very differently about art, ceremony, livelihood, and the social fabric? Why not about religion, too?

It takes a long time to give up wanting to beat the prison guards of rationalism at their own game. But when confronting the challenges of our myriad global crises, here's a good question: Would ritual get the job of real change done? Or did it breed a different kind of addiction, so that one developed a need for the energy that was only forthcoming in a circle breathing deep? Maia said it didn't matter—thoughts have power. In a tight spot she put beings in all the four quarters, regardless of whether she was being arrested in a nuclear weapons blockade or applying for a coveted job.

✳ ✳ ✳

All too soon it was time for the camp's grand finale. The work would be intensely personal, a complement to the lives to be lived after the Cadre's magic was done.

Cedar Wing and company knew there was an inner saboteur inside each of us, a perennial critic, nasty and overruling. It was a self-hating bugger, born of a finger-pointing parent, public schoolteacher, or a minister-priest behind the scene. But the Cadre dared to suggest that it had a deeper root. They called this saboteur the Inquisitor, and on our last night at camp we were invited to oust it for good.

The build-up began during our last afternoon. We were freed from the structured class schedule to go hunt for a vessel for the Inquisitor's demise. Playing hooky felt good—we were so used to a rhythm after two weeks of casting circles, moving energy, singing our throats dry, and wearing down the pine-needle floors with many a spiral dance. Alone or in small groups, we wandered the acres of Juggernaut Farm or sprinted across the coast highway to the headlands, the sea. We were on the lookout for a symbol, a carrier, any humble item to represent the Inquisitor so that we could demote that bastard in the flames.

They burned witches, didn't they? Now it was time for a symbolic about-face. I heard it time and again at camp: women spoke with an unhappy certainty about a past incarnation during The Burning Times, the Inquisition's search-and-destroy of all things female, of nature, of those listening to a different drummer. Though it was only history now, it was clear that even within the campers there persisted fear of a wild, natural self and all the trouble she could make. Today the inner Inquisitor was a lone terrorist, with the Vatican's implicit backing, who still held the same, deprecating views. Hence the upcoming ritual of purification: the flames of campfire would break the chains.

Walking along Juggernaut Farm's trails, I couldn't believe I'd be leaving the next day. I stood where chilly Northern California waves gifted the air with a scent entirely missing in Kansas: seaweed mixed with salt water and sand. So much else about this place and time would never translate. How would such precious soul-cargo survive the plane ride home? Should I stay here?

Yet back home was *home*. I was too prairie-rooted to reverse time. Where else could I rattle around in a house, visit a pond, and raise my arms to the moon with so much space to myself?

And there was the problem of my novice status. The older camp women possessed a confidence and abandon I lacked, though I was gaining on it. I wanted to be like them, especially Cedar Wing—what a pipe dream. Once away from Juggernaut Farm I would long for the smooth Flint Hills in part because, for better and for worse, it was where I belonged.

There was no whiff of evangelism about the camping witches beside the sea. Any hint of such thing was frowned upon, too much like You-Know-Who, the Christians we were careful not to mention. If I had a natural curiosity about finding like minds at home, it was for the sake of kindred rather than to (shudder) spread "beliefs."

Without a doubt I was profoundly put together anew by this experience. "Transformation" was the camp buzzword. Every day, when the confines of my tiny tent filtered the first light, I marveled at the Goddess, the tools, the way redwoods in fog were a portal to worlds that not only soothed me but in which I participated at the ground level. I had spent so many years without all this.

But the Inquisitor was still operative within. I knew it in the way I watched Cedar Wing paint a perfect crescent moon on her forehead on the last day of Camp. To me, everything she did was perfect. So what if Maia pandered to Griffin, Bloudewedd was snippy, Athena was openly insecure, and Ravenstar put raisins in every dish? Cedar Wing kept her cool for two weeks in a group of forty men and women emoting, changing, doubting, and challenging. She was an authentic priestess of the Goddess, and I'd never met one before. Now I had.

Get thee behind me

Thus an uptight rationalist like me fell for the whole thing hook, line, and sinker. Sure, I was coached by Chris Glen to lean left and care about the oppressed. That's probably why I trusted Cedar Wing. When she got fanciful with iron pentagrams and pulverized shark's teeth, it was firmly grounded in a wider vision. In the very next sentence she'd talked about how the witches had energized a feminist march against pornography. In the sixties occult world, this would have been unheard of. With the "leftist" and "alternative" folk exhausted and rudderless by the mid-eighties, the argument against imbibing spirituality with your politics had fizzled. Cedar Wing and her kind were everywhere, infusing nonviolent direct action with—there's that word again—*power*, a deep well for one and all. Power re-visioned as a force not to be wielded over others, but shared. That kind of power encompassed, but didn't stop at, acting solely on one's behalf. Thank Goddess it was all right to want and to have *power* again.

The campers discussed all of this at length, dissecting themselves and each other. How perhaps my Catholic girlhood, with its pomp and ceremony, had laid a favorable seedbed for ritual—even if in the pews I was bored stiff. Or, as the daughter of a professor, they suggested, maybe your mother and father gave you a love of books that prepared you to go overboard about the great ones. (At which Cedar Wing blushed.)

I wondered if we all had an innate predisposition to quest—was there a genetics common to searchers? Privately, I was priming myself for a startling thought about the Wohler Madness, a less than powerfull inheritance.

As with the moon's first words to my mind in the Flint Hills, the camp experience presented yet another dimension where issues of madness and sanity were not just relative, but irrelevant. Transcended, even. Many of us struggled, even in the circle, with our "stuff." But why did we seem to break loose so fast from wallowing and rumination into insight? The simple act of sitting in a circle—versus the doctor and patient face-off—replaced potential abuse of authority with equality. Cedar Wing, along with some of the other teachers and a few of the attendees, even possessed legitimate therapist credentials. But there was a refreshing freedom from that kind of jargon. Mostly, I think the healing was accomplished by the leap from the intellect—and one's personal problems—as supreme reality to a lived understanding that our church was the woods, the deserted cove beneath the headlands, and each other.

Or did the camp mesmerize us because the Cadre had a cloistered and consenting audience upon which to manipulate layers of consciousness? Maia met that remark with her finest witch's cackle.

Then why did I need so much time alone, striding back to the tent between activities to stare at the walls of my maroon cocoon? The Cadre would say that magic was tiring work. In time I'd find another answer. Despite the smiles and gentle ways, I made no lasting connections with any of the women there—I only endlessly compared myself to them. And I painfully watched myself doing so, which made matters worse. So as I scouted the grass along the headlands and thought about my self-hater, I was keen for a symbol of the inner meanie who insisted that I immerse myself in others to find out who I was.

Clambering down to the beach, my eye caught on a strange Earth sculpture barely hanging onto the soil: a mass of root, weathered from the ground, an easy handful of tangled gray-brown. It was a claw with uselessly skewed tentacles, misshapen through improper contact with the elements it craved. Not yet driftwood, but too exposed to ever heal into the Earth again, the root pulled easily out of the slope where it hung by a dry thread. Precisely! A picture of my Inquisitor's nasty disposition.

It wasn't the root ball's fault that erosion of the headlands had ripped it from home while all it ever wanted to do was grow in the sun. What had purpose in soil shriveled in winds it was too tender to meet and survive. Just so the critical voices within: initially helpful, cautious guides, they could warp into one big spoiler. In medieval times, every hack working for the Inquisition had a legitimate career before he was appointed witchfinder.

All the same, it had to go. Because, as the Cadre instructed, the self-hating voice carped, stalled, and spat: it stood between you and Power. So at the hour of midnight, the camp members dressed in their finest robes and trekked to the circle outdoors. Cedar Wing took up the drumbeat to cast the Inquisitors down.

We became trees, then, for the last time in this sandy soil. Roots down, branches up. We turned for one last look to the East, and it was Cedar Wing in fine form, a herald on intimate terms with the night:

"Welcome again, you Spirits of Air, we ask that you send winds to scatter all doubts as we prepare to step back into the world. With your bright new dawn we'll move every witch way (giggles) across this country to begin once more. May the magic of your crystal-clear power to *discern* be always with us."

Then Athena spoke with trembling voice and we were with her, turning our bodies to face the south: "Ancient Watchtowers of Blue Faerie Fire, we burn with you. We burn for knowledge, we are sparks in the force that drives the world to create and re-create. With your flames, we light our lives. Be with us—here, tomorrow, and always—when we seek energy, belly laughs, passion, and more!"

Another quarter-turn, and the headlands were out there. The waves seemed in sync with our hearts. "Mighty...deep...swelling... birthing waters of the West," began Maia, sounding male in register when she pitched it so low. "We feel you. We surf. Now that we trance and lovingly spiral dance, these good Witches of the West take from you a new place to travel—between worlds. Let compassion be the bridge between everyday land and limitless sea."

Ravenstar, our cook and herb magician, was dressed for the occasion. He was the archetypal Green Man in velvet and silks, emerald and gold flashing in the firelight. Brown as a walnut trunk, he swayed to the North, waved, leaped, and shouted words in Swahili I didn't understand. Then he collapsed into a heap. All were silent. Slowly he unwound: a finger, a foot, limbs uncurling into the night. Back from his trance, he smiled wide: "Spirits of Earth are definitely here, and want to follow everyone home."

Then the whole camp exploded with names, bringing their Goddesses and Gods back to life again through invocation and evocation. It was what we'd done every night, followed by chant and dance. The words were about power, but the net effect was pure joy. Cedar Wing's watchful eyes scanned the group, gauging our moment to shift, and then she began the wordless chant that built around and above those gathered. We sent it peak-first into the sky. She bade us sit or lie down and do whatever we would do with our eyes for trance.

"Linger a moment and touch this ground, remember all you have learned in these weeks, ready to take with you. Linger first in that place of peace where protection surrounds you, that place inside you've visited time and again when we work. Take the gift from whichever element—air, fire, water, earth—the Goddess hands you. Hold it tight for the last journey we'll make here tonight…a difficult one. We are heading back to a very sad time, centuries ago."

Her drum was steady, portentous. Our breathing was audible.

"If there are any special guides you need, gather them now to your vision; the vessel is here to take us between the worlds. A boat appears; it pushes through the mists, the eras drawn back before the birth of our grandmothers. Sailing backward go our souls. Grief was the daily bread when Inquisitors roamed the lands, looking for our kind."

She paused. A current of fear held the group; you could feel it in the dark behind your eyelids. You could also feel that we were resolute.

"We have landed. The countryside is a forest of burning stakes. All are under suspicion. You know this, you have been here before. But this time you are safe, you are a visitor, and as much as you'd like to enlighten the masses, the timeline cannot be disturbed. These centuries stand as a blight on history.

"Go now where your instincts lead. The seed of the self-hatred you carry to this day was not born here. Hatred of woman and Nature preceded the Inquisitors' torture. But here, in this sad time, the weeds grew berserk, unchecked.

"See now the witchfinder; see the malice in his eye. Malice especially for you and yours—your friends, your animals, the herbs grown outside your cottage door. He despises everything about you and is ready to render you to strange instruments that will inflict great pain. Finally the scaffold, or the fire. Listen to what he says."

The silence was heavy between drumbeats. A log shifted on the fire with a thud. We were left for a minute or two in an encounter with the king of the self-haters, personified.

"Breathe deep. Pull in power from the Earth, the Mother's breast still beating deep under the ashes of oppression. Now answer the witchfinder. Stare him in the eye.

"You know what you have to do. Find your power. Look closely at the Inquisitor: body, dress, and mannerisms. Look so close you can see yourself reflected in those cold eyes—and then begin, before all is lost. You have the power to change what was done. Say what you need to. The Earth is calling, 'Fight for me!' The trees are wailing, 'We will no longer give our wood up for fodder!' The very air cries, 'The smoke is so acrid the songbirds choke!' Fight for *them*."

Much weeping among the assembled. A few were writhing on the ground, rolling away from the fire as if it were their imminent destination. I heard Cadre members move near those most afflicted. As for me, I was awash in a mix of exhilaration and dismay.

At first, in mind's eye, I had indulged in a rakish Amazon battle and escape. Then following Cedar Wing's suggestion to look closer, I saw a parade of all-too-contemporary and definitely male naysayers. The father, the teachers, doctors, uncles, boyfriends, husbands…all the distant men who controlled me in the name of love, sneered at my rebellion, rejected my fire—or, worse yet, never noticed. There I was again, looking for their approval so that I could live and breathe. One tear made a beeline through glitter for the ground, but I was okay. Best to let the Cadre care for those in real trouble.

"Now you see what has changed. How does the Inquisitor appear now? What peace can you make with each other—is it even possible? It might not be. But is there a gift now in this whole turn of events, some lasting memento of transformation?"

She drummed and spoke no more. It took several minutes for people to get hold of themselves. Once the Cadre had decompressed the situation, you could almost detect a sigh in Cedar Wing's trance-voice.

"So it's time for goodbyes. Find your way back to the boat that travels the eras and come back to our time and this place. See on your journey home how the landscape has changed. Sail to your place of peace to rest and recharge. When you're ready, bring your eyes back to this welcoming and witch-friendly fire."

Cedar Wing drummed on intensely, insistently, winding about our crumpled and contemplative selves. Stirring us like a cauldron that had just boiled over, ripe for the last ingredient. Cadre members stoked the embers into a blinding blaze.

"You have an object. Do you wish to put it into the fire—not from hate or fear, but in service of change? Put your hand on it, take one last look. You share power now; stories of domination are no longer told between you. Hold this symbol of what once was, touch it one last time. Then advance to the flames and make the transformation complete."

People rose stiffly to regard the only light in sight. Into that heat went bits of private monsters—inner judges, juries, and executioners—invested with the soul-grime of lives lived under wraps. The witches were striding out of the broom closet, turning the tables as if to say, "With love, signed: the Goddess."

Into the fire they threw chips of marred shell, stones of all shapes and sizes, leaves marked with sigils of pain, and one crafty crown of thorns. Some campers simply hissed at the flames, or shrieked hateful names they wished never to hear again. In went my gnarled root mass, which stayed dull for a moment, as if immune, until the heat overpowered it into a dying orange.

"After all," Cedar Wing would say the next morning, "catharsis is our middle name."

Around this laden fire we danced until spent, then drew near on our haunches, thinking private thoughts. Some of us glowed, gloated, or positively glittered. Others, it was plain to see, had just opened Pandora's Box.

For the novice from Kansas, a far deeper understanding of the Wohler Madness was born. Inquisitor: forerunner of the psychiatrist. Squelcher of magic. He who would burn the female soul, able to round up more bodies than a human father ever could, henchman of Our Father. Women, laboring under the memory and the contemporary re-enactments, were still burning the witch within.

Divine madness was a potent antidote. I had savored it, and survived. It wasn't like Yr, nor where Agnes or Samuel went, but the pearl of the paradox: madness that heals. At last, with no doubt, I knew who I was. Being born into my family was some cosmic prank. I'd found where I belonged, the tribe whose crest I would wear each day, in the shape of a silver pentacle at my throat, for years to come.

Chapter 7
THE GOOD GUIDES

After Pagan Boot Camp, I returned to a place devoid of mentors in magic. But visions of wild women and laidback men still danced in my head. I could circle with them just by closing my eyes. It was the witch's way.

Home in Kansas at the farm that wasn't, I peered at the floor of my living room. Was I really going to lie there while a tape played suggestions to relax and "journey"? A tape I had to record myself? Would it be as good as Cedar Wing and Company in the flesh? These were skills I'd have to practice alone for now.

At the Camp by the sea, I took a big step from rationalist to ritualist in order to probe with the eyes of the mind. Now there was another minor leap ahead: forgo self-consciousness about the sound of my own voice. I'd have to talk to myself in a way that was neither poem nor conversation, nor persuasive speech. The curriculum was cobbled from scratch in the language of trance.

It was easy to recall the instructions from Cedar Wing, gentler things than run-ins with the Inquisition. Bits like floating on a cloud, or a pentagram of posies rising over breakers at dawn. Pretty things, nature things, profound and timeless things. The point was to visualize, visualize, visualize—and I hoped to sink like a stone. It was easy to pretend the head witches were in the room egging me on to "see" in living color, to ride breath to other planes as real as this paint-peeling parlor set amidst soybean acres and cattle plains.

Scattered on the floor were the essential books, all by women. How could I have missed this genre? These were not the hypnosis scripts of a profession keen to stop smoking, manage pain, or lose weight. Women were writing trance trips to sparkling, comforting, challenging, and scary places, to courageous and compassionate places, all because magic was ours. No more "for adepts only." The techniques were open secrets and ours for the taking.

At Boot Camp I'd heard the word "shaman" a lot, a figure synonymous with "medicine man" (or woman). I sensed that Cedar Wing felt she was in their league. So in my rough farmhouse in Kansas, I plunged into a study of shamanism in cultures where visits to spirit-worlds were a source of knowledge. At the heart of indigenous wise women's and men's healing abilities was the purported ability to travel for miles without moving a muscle. I looked around for an experience that might compare.

In Osage End, there was a slow wave of interest in sweat lodges. I wasn't comfortable plucking Native American techniques off the shelf, as if all were forgiven. It was not, and many contemporary shamans on this continent frowned upon the plundering of their mysteries. Still, there were universal components to the shamanic trance. Add in the Goddess flavor, plus poetic license aplenty, and voilà—a newborn technology of the sacred. I trusted my sister-spirits would create wisely, guided by their intuition.

Trance was the vehicle for a platform to other worlds after invocations to the elements of air, fire, water, and earth were called, the circle "cast." These were critical preliminaries—then came the story. The story was all bones, but strong bones. You met yourself where you could. The trance had purpose, substance, body. You went in like a miner of imagination after the nugget, and sometimes hit a life-changing vein of gold.

Far more exciting than the predictable inwardness of marijuana bliss, much like the moon talking to the simple point, what I heard in trance made sense. Rare but there, the shimmer of divinity was green at the heart and felt like an opening at the top of my head. On the floor, with no human ear within range, I propped pillows in appropriate places and hoped against hope to lose my body.

It's easy to see why I took to trance. Plenty of inwardness marked the predilections of my immediate family (minus my very social mother, whose solitary hours seemed to breed more self-pity than the strange relief the rest of us got from reverie). We spent so much time in our minds, tossing between great ideas and spinning scenarios of getting the best of everybody. Narcissus' stories always illustrated the art of coming out on top. Sam spoke of stalking a new mathematical theory in such a way that you knew it was attended by fantasies of how someday he'd be noticed, in a big way. I lost a lot of time to the same kind of daydreams. At the heart of it, for us, was this: someday, someone would understand.

If I could allow Cedar Wing and the Cadre to coax my mind into the middle of the Burning Times, could I revisit my own brush with the psychiatric Inquisition? What would the great rebels against that establishment have to say?

It took me a long time, after my comfortable friend among the B-Brothers told me to check out Thomas Szasz, but finally I did. I found that this Professor Emeritus of Psychiatry professed a lot more than "mental illness doesn't exist." He made the point that there was no gap in historical time between the winding down of the witch-hunts and the gearing up of the mental health establishment. What a frightening similarity in civil procedures: the automatic presumption of mental illness, validated by the claims of others, with involuntary confinements and "treatments" borrowed from the Inquisition. One hunt traded for another.

Seen in this light, the labeling of ever-younger people as disturbed and drug-worthy speaks about more than the need to help them. Drugs to a young, developing brain are double roulette—though not one doctor batted an eye at prescribing them to the Habitat hippies in 1969.

As a juvenile and a runaway, I'd had no rights to begin with. To stray so far from the norm as to forsake my good middle-class home… I must have been crazy. Those six months left an indelible mark, a tendency to forever look over my shoulder for the proverbial white coats. The *how could you?* of the Habitat staff was echoed for the benefit of our parents. We weren't treated as crazy so much as incorrigible kids. That was the ruse none but us could see through.

No, we didn't endure electroshock, lobotomy, or insulin coma at the Habitat. But the stigma fueled the same authoritarian sleight-of-hand—verbal taunts and insults with no real listening, because our words were the froth of a sick mind. This kind of abuse was far more contemporary, a chemical straightjacket for kids so out of control they found themselves within mental hospital walls.

To justify a profession's wages, we were deprived of free agency with a diagnosis that would haunt forever, and then shuttled through a palette of pharmaceuticals and impotent therapies because no one could figure out what else to do with such wretched youngsters.

The sham of being boarded up in such a place for so-called healing was easy to see through. As a (formerly) good girl from a good family, I had a certain amount of fun being bad. But years down the road, it hits you. You are marked by those outside who still believe heartily in the devil of insanity.

After my trance run-in with the Inquisition, with my fellow Boot Campers taking on similar villains, I distanced myself from the marks of psychiatry by leaps and bounds. I'd been steered into a nuthouse because my wild soul was unseen, or a threat. Good thing I didn't dabble in the so-called occult inside the Habitat—it would have only magnified the presumption of delusion, disease. I was already female and uppity (crazy) enough to sneak off from home and school, with the intent of disappearing forever. Thankfully, the Moon waited to speak to me at the edge of a field where She and I could be alone. If I'd only been able to hear her then, would She have changed me so radically that I'd have walked free of the Habitat in days?

Now, after all that, here I sat on my own hardwood floor, alone with a tape recorder and a little pointy microphone in hand, ready to record. Ready to surrender the conscious will. What I knew was that I was determined to kick out all the witchfinders who'd been eating my soul alive with a depression and anxiety so fierce that it plaited my dreams and blunted my ability to act.

Fifteen years post-Habitat, and only now could I consider anything as non-rational as spirituality or trance for fear of crazy-labeling. After my weeks at Camp, I had no desire to dwell on the mental health authorities' misdiagnoses of juveniles in the turbulent sixties. In fact, I felt I understood why I'd been delivered up to the place—not that I liked it. I was wild and witchy, a woman with a truth. *Narcissus had me scared to death.* My father, however, had handed me over to others to fix and those Habitat jailers were still within. They were the ones I needed to de-activate.

But first, practice. Gritting my teeth against self-consciousness, my own voice invited me to imagine a soft rain of healing stars sifting down. My mind wandered to my father's life. Could I say that his broken heart was fixed? He was *recovered*, had been for years. But he never went back to his old self-at-large. He and my mother had one childless couple with whom they were fast friends. In the company of this dyad, they tried to forget our family failures.

As I started to drift from awareness of the hard floor beneath me, I realized there was finally something bigger than this worn-out drama. I'd lucked into a juicy stay at Juggernaut Farm that cracked the world open, almost like traveling to a foreign culture. I found a history that linked madness and the Earth, and there were new ways of relating to beings that I had never met before. With some discretion I could pursue these trains of thought without raising the eyebrows of the ever-watchful—and largely rationalist—mental health system.

First, the good down-home stress relief of breath done to progressive relaxation, the sights and sounds of eyelid movies when I just let go. I was ready to race light years away. Without question, the "place of power" that the script instructed me to envision was, if not remote, then non-corporeal.

And the figures that populated these places—who knew I would be attended by so many "guides"? Were they real? What was the difference between this experience and Yr? Loving and tender and squarely on my side, if these guiding voices had spewed gibberish or urged harm I'd have scoffed and sat right up. But they were so straightforward with their "advice."

Animals showed themselves first: the deer, a crow, a coyote trotting by with a smile on his face. I brought them my problems and they showed or said what was possible. Or they ran into the woods, leaving me without a clue.

In later forays on the floor, persons with purpose showed themselves from within. An old lady lithe in white crinoline. A gardener whose plants grew out of his skin. But mostly goddesses: Artemis of ancient Greece, Bridgit of the Celts, and Ishtar of Sumer. And earlier icons of the naturally naked and faceless "fertility goddesses" from long before the marble temples where Greco-Roman priests split Her into specialties, precincts, jealousies.

I'd rise, shut off the tape player, eat and roam outside, then take to the floor again. This went on for three months, floated by the last of my student loan money for the semester. To my parents, I said I was studying the job market. Indeed. What needed studying was the entrance to this place of wonder that was shaping up as the finest insurance against the Wohler Madness that time could buy.

This imagining finally allowed self-supporting images and voices to triumph, dissolving the family disease on its own potential territory through the dance of trance-pictures on a farmhouse floor, in the hands of good guides.

✳ ✳ ✳

Looking for more resources on myth and ritual, I was excited to find the writings of John Weir Perry. Another brave psychiatrist chagrined by the drug-and-park-'em approach to mental illness, Perry posited that the chaos of the psychotic's world contains an ancient structure. He believed that if it were left to unfold—and patiently attended by a community of listeners—what looked like insanity would evolve into bearings regained and a wiser, more settled mind than before.

His premise was that schizophrenics could heal via the contents of their ramblings and visions, if only others would *hear* deeply and *honor* the mythological over the pharmacological. Instead of passing over such statements as the flotsam and jetsam of a disordered brain, Perry listened hard for the spiritual underpinning. He had the case stories to prove his method's viability, collected from a place of care he'd founded named Diabasis. Where else was it located but the People's Republic of San Francisco?

What if the protagonist of *I Never Promised You a Rose Garden* had Weir instead of Yr? The apocalyptic scenarios of his patients sounded so similar to Deborah's. Yet the girl's psychiatrist forced her to choose—in what became the last and final struggle of her journey—between her made-up fantasyland and the real world. No promises of roses if you decide to throw your weight with us here, but aren't your imaginary friends a bit immature? (True, they were vicious.) So at long last Deborah's inner kingdom dissipated. But it took her years upon years to let Yr go and to leave the hospital. Perry documented that if the "myth-styled" images of acute psychosis are properly handled, the troubled person returns to consensus reality transformed within a matter of days—six weeks at most.

Cedar Wing's grove beside the foaming headlands, with its night fires and dances, its afternoon student trances, healed a simmering volcano in me in just two weeks. But what about my older brother? Was Sam operating in a mythological landscape? Maybe something could be redeemed, maybe there was a bridge we could meet on. Maybe the Wohler Madness was a misnomer in more ways than in its bid for social control.

So I tried listening…deeper…to the content of my brother's paranoia. I wondered why he believed strangers in the supermarket line said things like, "Sam Elton is a shit!" Why did he sleep in our parents' house with a knife under his pillow? Why assert that a stranger in a café had slipped a "mickey" into his drink? What was the root of this perceived mass malevolence?

It was all about Sam. I tried but could hear no footfalls of the divine in Samuel's talk of others' evil doing towards him. I was straining for images of a mandala, wholeness, rebirth. But Sam was the aching, vivid locus of his and everyone else's world. I called him an egotist in private, a schizophrenic at large, reversing the tables to wear the contempt of the spiritual materialist. What a similar shuffle the Habitat staff had presented to its teenage charges: *Shame on your bad behavior…you poor thing!*

Another feature of Sam's plight-named-paranoid-schizophrenia was his enduring rage. Like father, *not* like son: Sam was never allowed to vent. After many trips to the hospital, he adopted a strange way of letting you know how angry he was and how he didn't agree with any part of you. It looked like some therapist had pointed out his stony visage and outright glare and urged him to do something about it. Sam's compliance was coupled with an eerie protest.

Heavily medicated, my brother's complexion was waxen. Saliva slipped from the corners of his mouth and he often reached up to pull at an eyelid with the heel of his hand. He spoke when spoken to in monosyllabic monotone, followed by the dead giveaway that he may have been prompted to learn: a fake smile dropped too fast, a quick, practiced, somewhat grotesque upturn of the lips, more grimace than grin. The motion expertly conveyed his underlying objection through the speed by which it was withdrawn. It said more than just *a therapist told me to act nice.* Maybe I was the paranoid one, but to an estranged sister it looked more like: *You worm, leave me alone.*

I gave up trying to visualize Sam on a spiritual quest, and focused on reconfiguring my own Habitat stay in light of trance discoveries. On the one hand, fifteen-year-olds shouldn't pursue drugs under the guise of countercultural ethics nor hitchhike hundreds of miles to Denver. To disappear for a month, to obsessively glue myself to anyone and everyone, to find my family so troublesome as to make me nauseous—had I been of clear mind, I might have applied brakes to this excess.

Yet at the time I just ran, thinking the Eltons and Osage End unhip, telling myself I was entitled to better. I felt unloved in the house where I was forced to live, invisible at school and in my small hometown, but that was too scary to face. The quest for freedom in all things was a grander flag to wave.

In time I faced squarely what really drove me away: the family's belief that my antics, left unchecked, would kill my father. But in 1969 my actions coincided with Agnes' empty shoes to fill: the Wohler Madness explained the unexplainable. So my father knew where to place me when I stepped so far over the line he could confirm that I was hellbent on murder. It was either him or me.

When he admitted he was out of his league and started searching for a solution that could be bought, the same stripe of man who once handled Agnes was quietly called one evening. *I can help you,* said a colleague familiar with the discipline of psychiatry, familiar with the Great Plains Mental Health Habitat. This was the kind of "help" that men still give women today. After all, witch-hunters and whole villages burned to drive out the devil have long been too untidy for educated persons to bear.

Today, they only fry the spirit.

It was one thing to shoulder adolescence as the black sheep. It was another thing altogether to be branded the cause of my father's heart disease. I had my life ahead of me, but he had a more important one ongoing. Apparently I believed that too, and did the family a favor by leaving: first for Denver, then for the Habitat, then by marrying Chris Glen so ridiculously young.

One month past Boot Camp, I was under a moon shining hard and bright. A quality of all this trance work was emerging: it made me more truthful with myself. So I let myself go back to 1969, eyes wide open and ready to hurt. I dared to ask the Moon what if—at fifteen, and free—I had never been found, in the mountains or anywhere else?

Once, while hitchhiking in Denver, a man grabbed for me as I slid out of his car. I didn't think about how lucky I was, only *what an asshole!* I refused to believe hitchhiking might get me on the wrong side of a dangerously strange ranger. The freeway ramps were surely lined with my kind because drivers were nice, and happy to have company in their cars. We, the recipients of their generosity, were the embodiment of freedom and love, so they should be thrilled to have us.

Yes, but. I never faced how badly things were headed. Three days before the Denver police came kicking down the door, I was being persuaded by my new friends, some speed freaks, to put a needle into my arm. They'd asked me about it, if I'd ever wanted to shoot speed. When I fervently spoke of hating needles, the headman smiled sweetly to himself. "You will," he said, "want to in time."

The memory still made me shudder, even years later under Her light and utterly protected within the silence of the prairie undulating for miles. "Dammit, I was an innocent kid from Kansas with a smart mouth," I told the Moon. "I didn't know how to ask You to watch out for me. Had I known, I probably would not have run."

It was a monumental shift, a dropped guard. It happened between Her and me first, though admitting it to another human being would come much later. Between my spirit and me, a most important wall came down when I admitted, "Maybe it was for the best that I was stopped in my tracks in Denver."

I only wished they'd found some other way than a nuthouse to derail me.

✳ ✳ ✳

Each day, as my sacred landscape shifted inside (and outside), I revised old stories in trance à la the Cedar Wing finale, finally draining the wounds. Then out of the house for what lay beyond: wildlife sightings, the cottonwood leaves' rustling prayer, a sunset spread orange and wide over the shoulders of the Flint Hills. The companionable creatures and features of the night were my touchstone. Why did it take me so long to absorb the full impact of earth and sky, beyond *it's pretty*?

I began to think about what estrangement from the natural world had done to my family. Outside the house, the lawn was an annoying chore. We beheld Mother Nature only on vacation. My parents preferred cities for their getaways, but in the summer they needed water and cruised the Lake of the Ozarks in a loud motorboat. A nice family and Nature: sunburned and suburban, trafficking the places made for tourists. Such a common story.

I never stopped tromping around outdoors as kids did before computers and sexual predators drew them inside. I could salve hurt feelings from peers and adults alike anywhere developers hadn't slashed the land. Interwoven with real leaves under cumulus towers, my daydreams outdoors were always more fruitful than hunkering inside standard-size bedrooms. Maybe this is why I ultimately escaped. The natural world, as my first therapist, gave me a fighting chance.

Now thirty-something, stalking visions with shape-shifting guides in trance, then rising to go outside and kiss my hand to the moon—it felt less crazy every day. There was continuity between nature in trance and walking the Flint Hills. I was being molded in ways that overshadowed the babble of the therapist's room, but how was I, how could I, keep this all to myself?

Time with my spirit guides brought new urges to the fore—and convinced me to end the standoff between school versus work. My immunity from the family disease was in the bag. I couldn't sit on what I knew about inner and outer landscapes dissolving the self-hater, and more. Could others be helped, as I had been, by the moon and Her many worshippers? Politics was no longer enough; there was more to madness than a ploy to squelch the downtrodden. I felt called to service in a way that only courting the divine can do. At last I was no longer the runaway, the pissed-off politico, an Elton-in-exile.

There was that word again, the one the Goddess women used: priestess. It gave me goose bumps in a way that "shaman" never did. I knew I wasn't one yet, whatever it truly was, and maybe I'd never be one. Priestess. Just a woman, but what a woman one could be.

Chapter 8
SQUARING THE CIRCLE IN THE MIND

I knew what I had to do. Just as I'd sought out pagan folk, I needed to know more about trance. I'd gone the distance with my floor time as far as an amateur could.

Once again I trekked to the west coast, to a California retreat quite unlike the witches' foggy lair by the sea. Well-heeled New Agers assembled in the heart of wine country. Highway 101, a major freeway, skimmed the hill just above our building, the swish of traffic with us day and night.

My fellow seekers were a different stripe than the magic-and-nature boot campers. Their preoccupations were with "Light" and other incomplete concepts recycled from stressful religious upbringings. Plus money. They came to learn how to make more of it. None would be caught dead calling themselves "political," let alone pagan.

Our fearless leader was a squirrel-like, self-styled master who melded his take on shamanism with the best of the human potential therapies. He created a program that led me to the most powerful guides yet. Even though Squirrel (as I fondly and privately called him) had some very annoying mannerisms, it was clear he was onto something.

Instructors gave us the formal tools of hypnotherapy in a highly structured course that covered the basics: how to get your client to the subconscious and how to help when they were there. But we came for more than mechanics, and Squirrel delivered. We would learn how to transport persons to their own sources of wisdom within. Guides, guides, guides for all. Not only witchy women and cunning men—*everyone* was entitled.

The first guide we would meet, said Squirrel, was key to the work. I suspected that the crowd was poised to meet images of celestial figures, or perhaps indigenous elders. Probably some of them had to flip a U-turn in order to grasp Squirrel's foremost suggestion: listen carefully to a vulnerable-yet-honest slice of self. For most of us, it would be a relief to be introduced. Hesitations in check, everyone tranced down to meet a small person with a great deal to say.

Enter the part of psyche that Cedar Wing had called Younger One, assuring us that this was the real source of magic and truth. Squirrel called this guide the Inner Child. He led us to envision and embrace this tender thing, and to champion the Inner Child's true needs.

Abuse. Neglect. Incest. Back from trance, recounting battles on behalf of their inner child, many had clear-cut stories of force and violence. But trauma is trauma is trauma. Squirrel and his minions told us not to compare one gruesome growing-up with another. Being raised with Narcissus in the House of Paranoia was a lesson in how mistruth creates trauma. As the father-reviling rebel who caused the cardiac crisis, I never stood stand a chance. The Habitat was a foregone conclusion the minute I saw through the lies that kept this system in place. By then, my Little was scared out of sight.

In the innocence of my inner child, I discerned no tendency toward the Wohler Madness. Rather, in her simple basic wants and needs, I saw Every Girl. Within her very common yearnings for love and good times there was no speck of pathology, no demon child waiting in the wings. In trance I took her out of the Elton home, off the Wohler roster. What especially pleased me? I, who had avoided parenting so long due to fear of my capabilities, took to this task of parenting her with ease. She was a joy to have around.

The beauty of Inner Child exploration is that you are the one doing the redemptive work. You don't need a professional—although without Squirrel to provide a safe container crafted by his leadership, I doubt I could have embraced the younger self with such total love. Trancing down below the chattering rationalist also helped her to emerge. Squirrel emphasized that this guide was a gateway not to narcissism but to healthy self-love, even a route to the divine. I knew that this stuck child within never had an advocate, until the Goddess. Agnes' unconditional love was a close second.

Later, it would never cease to amaze me—the look of recognition on most faces when I spoke of inner child work during the period when it consumed me. Even when others resisted or pooh-poohed it, their discomfort said a lot. The child was alive enough to peek out through many a closed gate. Every adult knew there was suffering there, knew it in his or her bones and blood. Most who came to meet theirs did so with a mix of great fear and great willingness. It is instinctual to save a child. There are also ecstatic, stored memories of oneness with life that this guide holds. Yes, even those abused horribly from day one can recall such things.

I thought I'd be a "single parent," but not for long. Another day, another helper in store. Convened by Squirrel, we were told about another figure essential to reclaiming the inner child and keeping her safe. When it came to this guide, you saw much less trepidation and much more clear-cut interest among the hypnotherapists-to-be.

First, the buildup. It involved much talk about getting in touch with your Male Side (if you were a woman), or the Female Side for men. How only the Inner Family could wipe out the carried scars of the spirit. Gay people were acknowledged and allowed to choose a different gender mix for the family within.

Thinking about consorts and lovers of the Goddess, I wondered who might show. Then I decided it was best not to get too high-falutin.' This guide could have perfect love and steady wisdom, but he would essentially be a surprise. I didn't want to program in a myth that I was making up for me, although if it happened that way, fine.

Once again, we spread about the plush-carpeted floor and prepared to meet another parent for our inner child, the Inner Lover.

I thought back to the night before this important descent. I'd relaxed outside in a hot tub as shreds of dusk gathered below the freeway. Against the fog rolling in, I saw wings cut the sky: some kind of hawk, circling. Later I'd learn its name—osprey, not native to the Flint Hills of Kansas. The osprey dipped lower, circling the tub area, and cocked its head to look at me. Was there was a mouse running by my bubbling cauldron? The tub adjoined a swimming pool, with the whole area paved in concrete and ringed with cast-iron. Besides a flowerpot or two, the unnatural expanse reeked of chlorine. An unlikely hunting ground.

But the osprey was definitely looking at me. Streaks of light and dark brushed his torso and wings. I could mark the slightest move of his head as he spiraled above. Like so many moments on the prairie, this one seemed to stop time.

Squirrel led us to find our soul's mate that next day. Always primed to pay attention to animal sightings, I wasn't ready for such a personal shifting of shape.

I saw the osprey's eyes. He said to follow him.

And, in that limitless way that is trance, I flew with him to a beach of boulders. Rocks piled for miles as if the moon touched down and left rubble behind. The osprey settled onto one of the larger stones and changed into a man—a very attractive man, although not my usual template of skinny blond longhair with a go-go attitude.

Big but not beefy, "Os" (as I'd later name him) wore a cassock much like a monk's, but tailored and lightweight as if to suggest taste over asceticism. His hair was dark, cut cleanly between long and short. We had our first talk about my problem with relationships.

He knew what I'd been through, hopping from heart to heart and into heartless beds along the way. Though we were being guided by our trance-guru, trusting this vision came effortlessly. Most importantly, he was there not only for me, but also for Younger One. She accepted him without reservation.

We were three then, and thanks to Cedar Wing the number was not lost on me: complete. Judging by the sniffles I heard, I knew that many memorable moments like mine were occurring around me. It was such a different kind of catharsis than the drum-trances at Camp. If Cedar Wing was all about taking back power, this exercise was a sure bet to reclaim love.

Talking to Os was a great deal like talking to the Moon, but a bit more like a blossoming romance. It was okay to fall in love with yourself this way, Squirrel assured us during the recap, explaining the anima/animus, a Jungian idea about the hermaphroditism of the soul.

You had to balance 'em, he said, your guy and your gal within. He also coached us on the differences between the inner lover and the outer relationship. Only coincidentally, he told us, did his actual wife and his inner woman bear the same name.

After this, I found myself squinting and frowning less at Squirrel for his political incorrectness. I had to hand it to him: he gave me the keys to Younger One and set the stage so I might bond with Os, who liked best of all to tell me: *You too can do what I do.*

Squirrel cautioned us that these techniques were "not for the psychotic." Aha! Again, a clear demarcation between the family disease and myself. We could tell a good guide from the monsters of Yr. We could get better, while psychotics could not. Those lost souls were left out of the New Age altogether.

It was fine by me, and with Os' help I contemplated becoming a healer like him. In further sessions with my inner lover I saw that he lived near the beach of bosomy boulders, in a hobbit-like house where he received the troubles of the community and healed them with hands-on energy work. And talk, and trance. He was a role model, and there were many men and women at the training who worked like him. Could I do the same? At least I wouldn't have to deal with the black holes in a person like my brother. I had permission only to share what I'd learned, to link up seekers with their inner child, their inner guides. But the boundaries were clear: *for neurotics only.*

I didn't have to save Sam.

And I'd be forever protected. A therapist! Safe at last!

Priestess for hire

After a period of practicing on friends and acquaintances, I put out a shingle of sorts. I saw mostly young female undergraduates with sexual abuse issues or eating disorders. For these, I had been trained. *Not for psychotics.*

The work dovetailed with the gaggle of students and alternative-types drawn to pagan ritual. We gathered at the solstices, equinoxes, and old Celtic holydays in between to merge lightweight therapy and even lighter devotion to the gods. Our rituals implored the forces of nature to help us with our problems. As with most religions' stock-in-trade, the celebrant hopes to harvest something from the otherworld to apply to nitty-gritty life. Trance: I led a few in the Circle, much like in the therapy room.

One of the things that set us apart from the love-and-light New Agers was our fondness for discovered old ways—not just in celebrating earth, but in trying to climb inside the ancients' minds. Due to Friedrich Wohler's ghostly presence I found myself drawn to alchemy, the forerunner of modern chemistry. It was something that also laced Squirrel's metaphors of change and transformation.

I approached alchemy with a modern disdain for the barely technological. Surely it was a practice for gullible souls trying, literally, to turn lead into gold with all manner of distillation and cogitation. I found that, while hucksters and simpletons were present as they were in any endeavor, there was more. Alchemy had a spiritual side.

The lead was the lazy, greedy, unaware self, bungling through a day, a life. The gold that the alchemist sought to make out of plain lead stood for enlightenment. Squaring the circle was one of my favorite alchemical symbols. It took the impact of the Three and added one more interesting note. Squaring the circle meant aligning the Four: body, mind, spirit, and soul. Looking to each of the four directions, as in Cedar Wing's trainings, and weaving their lessons harmoniously. Squaring the circle meant you ended up with a sphere: wholeness. If madness was the ultimate fragmentation, then squaring the circle was the ultimate practice of health.

Why the Inquisition mostly left the alchemists alone is a good question. By and large, the seekers were men. There was plenty of imagery of the divine feminine in their work, but they weren't out and about being earthy and sensual, curing and creating community on the land. Nor were they poor and rural; these were educated men. What if many, in their time, believed that they just might succeed at making real gold bricks? Then everyone would be rich, and there was no speck of threat in that.

Nor were there any modern-day Inquisitors stalking the tribes that sought to resurrect a Western mystery tradition. We were thoroughly post-modern seekers marooned without a tradition, desperate for some type of Earth-honoring roots. Though Kansas may not have been the best location to be reborn as a witch, there was always the humorous figure of Glinda the Good from Oz to cite. Even Kansas college towns tolerate their harmless kooks, which is how our small band of pagan players got by with celebrating the old festivals of the earth in public parks. If the police showed up we calmly informed them about solstice or equinox, as if such ceremonies were the most natural thing in the world (and once, they were). The authorities accepted us and quickly departed; they'd been to seminars on how to differentiate maypoles and drums from the sick minds that used these sorts of trappings to harm.

Meanwhile, in my consulting room where Tarot cards, massage, or ceremony worked alongside hypnosis, I subscribed wholly to the near-religious notion of therapy as a "sacred container" for the work of the gods. Many of my contemporaries and I, high on experimental times when it seemed that the folk healer was returning, took our office so seriously that we were in danger of losing sight of an ethic that encompassed humility. Demi-goddesses, we floated above the clueless, and whenever a client tripped our trigger and gave us "something to work on," it was part of the divine plan.

At last I was Fringe Woman, a pagan priestess and counselor for the spirit, trained in techniques I didn't have to sell my soul to receive. And I was living the dream in a midsize, university town in the middle Midwest. To onlookers, an interesting curiosity. Inside the university, my kind was fodder for a few good laughs. If on occasion the stray academic visited the village witch, it was done entirely on the sly.

When you're busy, you don't think much about whether or not you fit in. You swim in a sea of reciprocity with comrades and clients, you avoid the mainstreams or, during unavoidable contact, silently stoke your sense of superiority. I managed my route through the world carefully.

As for the Wohler Madness, I had the tools to stay sane and a profession to prove I would never succumb. There was a very thin line between the teachings of Squirrel and Cedar Wing, and if they'd known each other they would have recognized this. Magic taught me the discipline to stop simply reacting to bad things and running away. Magic taught me to focus intent. Magic made me deepen the real nature of my desires and go after them. Magic was an avenue that ran in a different direction from impulse, yet exciting enough to permit delayed gratification.

I didn't pour out my troubles to the Moon so much anymore. Instead, I "invoked" countless ancient forms of Her name to aid me in my magical work, and counted on this support. Many targeted goals came into manifestation: a spiritual community, a chance to earn and be fulfilled at a unique form of work. I was smitten with magic, hooked on ritual. I made altars the way others made art.

The Goddess, I felt, looked on in approval. Not that I forbade the God, her consort or son, a place in my rituals—He was a cozy and welcome partner, like a divinely inspired relative of Os. I looked around our sacred circles and saw Him in the faces of men there. By assembling to celebrate and heal, I believed that we were repairing the split between women and men—in fact, we all felt that we were living our highest ideals. We bucked hierarchical religion. We were in the trenches, crafting something new where gender equality was the norm. We were healing the earth with our good intentions. Why then were so many of us—when it came to relationships—still such a mess?

Chapter 9
GATHERING BY THE WATER

Something about that bridge.

Crossing over the river, I left town for an expanse of mono-cropped grain that lay on either side. The bridge was a gate: I was forsaking people, gaining limbo, the farmhouse still a half-hour ahead. But that night, I wasn't ready for the bridge, nor for my silent (if enchanted) prairie home. I was done for the day, but I needed the river over which that bridge kept watch.

A swirl of dirt marked the parking lot frequented by fishermen on weekends and by nobody at dinner hour. Yesterday's rain was moving the water at high speed, not quite ready to swallow its own banks. I couldn't say why I needed this place, only that the river was raising its voice.

I recalled coming here as a teenager furious with pain. Gravely banks bore the stomp of my angry footsteps as I skimmed rocks into the brew below, dark with eroded topsoil. Two decades later, I was harboring another set of growing pains. I *thought* everything was okay. But someone else felt differently.

I picked a spot hidden from the short old bridge and its arches of lichen-stained concrete; what I didn't need, at that moment, was the thump-thud of the occasional crossing car, or someone seeing me acting like a madwoman, talking to myself. "It's all right—I've been trained to do this!" I called to the river. If there was anything that Squirrel had taught me, it was the power of the inner players to work out conflict. I had come to gather the Judge, Innerchild Little Sue, Rebel Girl, Beloved Os, plus other guides and saboteurs, and let them hammer it out. The irony of it always grabbed me: *I hear voices, but my brother is the one medicated for it.*

The need to allocate these conferences to a state of trance, while lying on my wood floors or snuggled in bed, was a fading necessity. I could feel my inner aspects, good guides, with me much of the time. We were a cozy lot; I trusted them. They could count on getting a hearing. It wasn't so much the river that needed to speak, I reflected, as I high-tailed it further from the bridge, the cars, and the town. It was the whole crew within.

The Judge stood up first, already a force of urgency in my skin. He walked to water's edge, turned back to where I sat along the bank, then frowned. When he wasn't carping, I appreciated his insights. Regardless, any time he took the podium everyone within tensed and stood ready to defend.

"What is the relevance of this spiritual journey of yours? It's been years since you did any real work for the oppressed. If you do march, it's with an ankh at your throat and magic on your mind. It's guess it's the Me Decade for Sue. Fun! So much easier for you."

That's just his way. Calling you on the carpet. After all, he is the Judge.

"What's wrong with fun?" the child asked, picking up a piece of river rock, uncertain of where to throw it. She often felt the Judge was more of a prosecutor than one who balanced the scales fairly.

Os was at the ready. "You're saying there's no validity in what she's become over these past years? That we aren't modeling a new view of what the oppressed could feel and do? Besides, there are convents and monasteries for contemplatives, but where does the Earth mystic fit?"

"Spare me the bliss-babble," the Judge snorted. "I'm glad to see the nature thing evolve into more than escape and supplication, but what happened to fighting the good fight?"

Rebel Girl whirled about to face the Judge. It was good to feel her fire. "We're doing that by being one with the Goddess. Energy spent re-establishing that connection will lead to the peace that once was—in *Her* Garden of Eden."

"You never answered my point about the mystic being denied in a secular society," Os pressed the Judge.

Rebel Girl: "Yeah, I guess it's okay for nature-lovers with expensive hiking boots to pony up dues to environmental groups, but for Pete's sake don't make a *religion* out of it!"

"Can *I* say something?" I asked. When the "I" spoke, it was often called the Higher Self, though I preferred Cedar Wing's more Earth-based term of Deep Self. "Look, the culture is shifting. There's an appreciation of free-form individualized spirituality—it goes beyond Me-ism. It's creative, collective—you gotta see that it *is* direct *action* to push through the borders of dogma. This is a real chance for spirituality, *not* religion, to take its place beside intellect. That's fighting the good fight, a very peaceful one. Any act of genuine searching is going to ripple outward if the courage is there to see all the implications through."

Everyone looked at me, wondering if that mouthful held more. But I felt spent, and knew that was the extent of Deep Self's wisdom.

The Judge started pacing. "It's that handful of problem *words* you use," he said. Maybe that was what had been bothering him all along.

The Judge's case
We all knew what words he meant.

He continued: "Pagan. Goddess. Priestess. Witch. There may be a 'new' American spirituality, but *those* words belong to its illegitimate children. People want to hear about 'Light'! Abundance! Prosperity! They want to rise up and get off the wheel of death and rebirth, not keep coming back to the bloody belly of this earth-plane, Mother or not. Preferably not. The Goddess is, well, too *sexual* for them, don't you think?"

I heard Os gasp—but really, the Judge wasn't a bad sort. I could see what he was pushing for. More legitimacy for our mission. Rethink the lexicon that freaks out the listener, terms that require so much explanation, that keep you looking over your shoulder for the fundamentalists who'll take offense.

The Judge tried to soften his plea. "Look, it's been all these years. I know who you are, who we are. I get the history lesson. It's just that... you're not going to be able to be so blatant someday. Have you ever thought of that? No, because you don't think about the mechanics of the future. Much as you like to say you've changed, you still just live for today, right? But you know you can't hide behind that fake-enlightenment forever."

The inner child shook as she gathered more rocks in a pile. Talking about the nuthouse was a low blow—and I knew she was also remembering Catholic school, daily mass, the gruesome cross and the martyrs' deaths. Were the Inquisitors really dead? When the Judge questioned how far we'd come, she was afraid we'd be going backward.

Os sat down beside her and told the Judge, "Now listen here, you. I am of the Mother. She gives me life. Her blood is sacred, and all pleasure and play in Her name are good."

I adored the man. It was one of the many times when I ached to behold him in the flesh. Yet despite the attentions from her father, Younger Sue fidgeted and picked at her fingernails. She was the barometer, the only truly authentic reading of these proceedings.

"Look, everybody." I rose to match the Judge's pacing, then walked in a circle as if to gather them all in. "A spiritual awakening like we had surpasses falling in love. You just don't fear rejection the same way ever again, so there's a tendency to do less rejecting. Let's don't polarize. She shines on all, even Inquisitors. Yep, even on the Elton family and every other parental unit that introduces havoc into a life. C'mon, years ago Cedar Wing and Squirrel handed over some powerful stuff that set the course for this adventure. It gave us the best-yet antidote to the family disease. We will think very, very carefully before we call what we are by any other names."

The Judge still wasn't satisfied. Everyone was frustrated.

I tried another appeal. "Your Honor, what troubles you? We need constructive criticism here. Haven't I, haven't we, slowed down and stopped running so much? Don't we help other people in the way we were helped? Don't we have a community of like minds, confused adult children though these new Pagans are? Didn't we leave the Wohler Madness eating our dust once we found out about the Female Divine, about magic? What could be wrong with the power to hear the voice of the land, the moon, that heron prowling the opposite shore?"

In my mind, the fact that She was She had come to seem less unique, more of an everyday acceptance, even though at rock bottom I could scarcely presume that Spirit had gender. But I wouldn't let go of the need for a deity who looked like me, one not far removed from the senses, who delighted in seasons, color, sustenance, and starlight.

Maybe the Earth as a holy place is creation the way we're trained *not* to grasp it. If I could sense this, I knew anyone could. I wished the Judge could see how pertinent it was that humans regain access to the natural world's chorus with its constant themes of beauty, vibrancy, and change.

I walked over to the rock where the Judge had chosen to hold court. One more step, and the murky river would be up to the knee. Standing perilously posed, I took him all the way in—and heard his objections take an abrupt turn.

Achilles' head

"It's just that you're not *completely* better," he mumbled. "What about the headaches?"

During the frequent migraines that took me out of commission, I felt vulnerable. That searing pain on one side of the brain was yet another family inheritance (both parents had them) for which there also seemed to be no cure.

"Headaches!" It was Os. "I take care of her when they happen."

"But she can't always trance down to you," the Judge objected.

He had me there. There were days at a time when I felt completely abandoned to the pain, and all I could do was wait.

Magic failed whenever frequent migraines came to visit, sometimes at hormone-raging moments but often out of the blue. Then blinds-drawn solitary confinement was the ritual—or more like jail. Whenever I tranced, going down to be with Os, the pain was held at bay. Awake and fully conscious, I was battered by the most critical, nasty side of the Judge and a few other hidden saboteurs.

Living from one migraine to the next was work. I savored the good days but increasingly felt ruled by the headaches' arrivals and departures. Still, I figured it was the lesser family curse. I grown up watching my mother succumb, and when Samuel and I were very little our father had taken an experimental drug—he never could remember the name of it—that had obliterated his for all time.

In the realm of migraine, I allowed my spirit to be crushed by resounding negative voices because it hurt too much to fight back. These voices didn't have faces, characters, or names. They were me being nasty to me. I never thought, *These are phantoms, these will subside.* Part of the migraine's power was delusion. Get real, it said, *this* is the truth: you are hopeless.

Such desperation was forever pitted against the gentler support of my guides. While stricken, I didn't know whom to believe. It was a lot like what I read about Yr.

I was convinced that the headaches were an omission of faith and trust in the Universe, a form of repressed memory or anger, or some other New Age failing translated into physical pain. Until I figured out exactly what I was repressing, those lost hours—or sometimes days—were reckoned as my just desserts for pieces of an unexamined life left languishing. But such insights never abated the pain in my head. The episodes had to run their unfathomable course.

"What can I say, your Honor? What is it you want?"

"Go see a doctor."

"Another one? Those drugs don't work, or they wipe me out."

"Get a scan, an MRI—something."

"This is hereditary. It's no tumor. Sometimes I just need to shut down. Do you have to berate me when I'm vulnerable?"

"Do you think it could be…the family disease?" the Judge asked.

I turned to Os for help but he and Little Sue were preoccupied. We had company.

Ancestor oblique

A stone's throw downstream, another part of my mind had formed itself as an angular man in midlife. A wavy mop of hair, craggy face, clothes from another century. He was intent on the river's edge, one moment picking up rocks with a practiced eye and putting those of interest into a knapsack, the next filling a flask with brown river water. He barely glanced at Os, but he looked kindly and beckoned to Little Sue.

"Uncle?" she asked.

"Just Friedrich," he replied.

The Judge stood open-mouthed as Rebel Girl and I hastened over. It was the first time I'd ever hosted an ancestor at a gathering like this. I didn't know I was even thinking about him. Someone was, however.

"Are you the scientist?" I asked.

He nodded and got down to business. "What's this dirty white foam here?" Friedrich pointed at the river. "It flows, it eddies…keeps moving, keeps coming…from where?"

"It's run-off. Are you—"?

"Yes, I'm Herr Wohler. Now tell me about 'run-off.'"

"Chemicals, like phosphates," I said.

"You should know about those—your discoveries paved the way for them," the Judge piped up, trying to ingratiate himself. He was the one among us who was most impressed by greatness, considering himself farthest from the clutches of the family disease.

"Chemicals from where?"

"The fields, farms. Insecticides, herbicides," I said. "Listen, we have a problem here, and I'm wondering if you came to help me?"

"I know you have a problem. I practiced as a medical doctor for several years."

"I get these headaches," I began.

"You must rest. Take laudanum, it'll calm your nerves. Try opium and lie down."

"Um, that stuff is illegal now. Besides, I am calm most of the time. In fact, that's what I do for a living—teach people how to be calm. Hypnosis—you know about it?"

Wohler laughed. "Freud and the subconscious! Very experimental, unsubstantiated."

The Judge cleared his throat. "Sir, we have a fly in the ointment. We have a dark pall that sickens us for days, for which we have no cure."

"The migraines just come on suddenly with no rhyme, no reason," I said. "Is there something in my past I'm not looking at?"

"This river's not healthy," pronounced Friedrich. "You came here for a reason, didn't you? What about this dirty foam?"

"What does that have to do with a migraine?"

Friedrich Wohler faced me squarely. I remembered the first time I told a chemistry student about my apparent relationship to the Victorian scientist. The guy photocopied a portrait from a textbook about great men of science and gave it to me. Above Wohler's unruly mop of hair he wrote *I see the resemblance—I think?* Why did he sound doubtful? Maybe, I thought, because this Wohler was so focused, so gentlemanly, so stable…not like a nutcase at all.

"I can't tell you the source of your pain," said Wohler. "I urge you only to never give up attempting to find that elusive cause. It's there, and you are correct: you've no more got a tumor than your mother or father did. Keep an open mind. Perhaps it's not what you think. The most astounding things are often revealed quite by accident."

And with that he laid a hand on Little Sue's head, nodded to everyone, and set off for the line of willows behind us.

"Wait!" I cried. "Were you schizophrenic?"

But Friedrich Wohler kept on walking, back to his own time when rivers ran clean.

Last Judge-ment

I wanted to discuss Wohler's visit, but the Judge did not. Somehow the incident emboldened him to take another bull by the horns. He (a part of me) hungered for genius that would wipe out all fears, doubts, pain, and heartache—and seeing Wohler, we all began to dream bigger.

Robert Elton had launched the longing early: *smarter than the average bear.* That was us, he often reminded his brood—but Narcissus had to be on speaking terms with doubt. Even Samuel, the Brain, doubted his way into a Thorazine haze. But the carrot on the glowing stick remained. If we were smart enough, all would be well.

So the Judge was out for reform, and he wanted it now. That critical but often discerning part of me demanded that every part of me live up to its potential! He saw me living a life too safe, sipping herbal tea and advising young women whose pain was all too familiar, planning rituals and watching the moon rise. He couldn't leave well enough alone.

I knew what was coming: he wanted to stomp the Not Smart out of me once and for all. To him, that was as frustrating as the days I spent lying in a darkened room with a migraine, fighting the self-hater tooth and nail. There was a behavior that even Os, though compassionate, admitted was foolish. The Judge rode shotgun while the others took a quiet backseat.

That hidden, fruitless loop in my life was known as "relationships." I was getting more and more disgusted with that revolving door and what came through it. There was no one who seemed able to go the distance with me, nor I with him. I didn't need to hash over this impasse one more time. So even before the Judge started taking me to task, I blurted out the truth.

"I want a child," I said.

Os gasped. Rebel Girl cursed a blue streak while Young Sue turned it over: does that mean a playmate, or a rival? The Judge was silent. Then slowly, I felt his mind—my mind at its most discerning—register a new flush of intrigue. I had to hand it to him: he could appreciate a novel approach to any problem.

I proceeded to make my case. "Haven't I raised my Inner Child well? Isn't Os the perfect parent, too? Haven't I faced, unraveled, worked through enough for now? Isn't the Wohler Madness a distant threat that will never come true here? Wouldn't my problem with men best be grappled with in the secure arena of a long-term commitment?"

Rebel Girl just shook her head, contemplating the end of her freedom. The Judge had no counter points. "Might just be the ticket," he said. "You are pushing forty. You'll really have to stop running if there is a spawn you're tied to. You'll have to give mighty thoughts to the future. This could take the coward right out of you. I like it."

Os knew I wanted to be partnered for life, despite two marriages down the drain. He was not opposed. But Rebel Girl complained about diving for another man to pull us out—only to find that he was drowning, too, and then wind up being stuck with him eternally as the father of my child. Os said to stop gauging my desires against what anyone else thinks, especially anti-psychiatry's disgust with the nuclear family. I reminded everyone that we probably wouldn't get anywhere with the health stuff if I didn't get off the fence on this one. What would pregnancy do? I'd heard it was a very different headspace, gained through the intensity of the body's transformation.

"Now, this isn't like taking Thorazine in the Habitat just to see what it does to your head," the Judge cautioned. "This is a new and tiny, defenseless person you're talking about!"

"I get that. I'm ready." Turning to Rebel Girl, I asked, "What really worries you? Hasn't footloose and freewheeling been done to death?" She wouldn't answer.

That night, as I lay next to a married man while his wife worked the graveyard shift at Osage End's busiest factory, I came to a crossroad in the deepest recesses of my Deeper Self. Rolling away quietly to put distance between us while he lightly snored, I dropped into a well that was so dark and wide that only the arms of the divine could catch me there. As a silent howl of entreaty filled that space, the plea that followed was desperately sincere.

Goddess, give me a sign.

PART THREE
LUNACY'S BODY

Chapter 10
COSMIC CHILD

The relationship between Os and the Inner Child worked magic so subliminal that when I realized I wanted a baby, my first urge was to suppress the notion. Squirrel taught that the Inner Family was the ultimate emotional refuge; no one mentioned the possibility that it might turn a confirmed "no kids!" person to the opposite frame of mind. Fear slowly evaporated when I saw there was more going on than ticking biology or the next lark. What hounded me was a wish to immerse beyond beliefs and postures—take a stab at *living it,* not just talking about it. *It* being the next step, the stage ahead, the dream least expected.

There was never any question about two prerequisites to the baby: a live, flesh-and-blood mate, and land.

The latter appeared on a ramble: fifty acres for sale that didn't look at all like the worn old Flint Hills. The place was rife with trees; a creek bubbled through oak and hickory woods where owl mating calls rang like roguish laughter at dusk. The woods hid wildlife so well it made discovery of animal tracks a joy, while the water was low and friendly with limestone seats for resting near mini-waterfalls. Former owners' fences were in serious disrepair, granting access through the topography where rocky ledges made stair steps to thickets of wild plum.

Goodbye to the difficulty of being "earth-based" without being directly in relationship to Earth. My rental place in the old Flint Hills would never spell permanence; there were memories that stung, plus the landlord's monthly need. I left that open space for the woods and creek to learn in the lap of my Mother, Nature, most fitting if I hoped to be a mother. When my parents heard the agenda, they gave money for the down payment with glee.

The Precious One Who Would Come could not be raised in town. There was too much my child might miss among streets and shows and frantic "activities." Never should she or he be deprived of the mysteries in meadows and ravines, in the four seasons turning without the buffer of urban artifice. I couldn't keep nature from a human as purely without guile as nature herself. The land that would become "ours" was found.

The man was part of the plan, too, and the day before we closed on the place we got married. I would never doubt this was the partner destined to know the child best, to weather the upheavals that her coming brought forth.

Partner in puzzle piecing

He had a funny first name for a Kansan. It was Kai (invariably, he had to spell it for both the curious and the bureaucratic). But a surname like Brinkhoff was familiar enough, even if the combination kept people guessing. Which he enjoyed.

When Kai Brinkhoff's mother was in Sweden, on her way to a divorce, she drenched herself in its culture. Knowing that she was headed back to America's high plains, she gave her baby boy a name that would always remind her of the time of her life. Back in Kansas, she groomed him to refuse the locals' farm overalls and look instead to the white collar, the red sports car, law school, and living in town. It wasn't so much *smarter than the average bear*. More like *get the hell out of here*.

We met when a lawyer was needed for our tribe to sort out a contract. Across the table over legal papers, Kai couldn't look at me. It didn't strike me as arrogance or disregard, but radar that communicated everything. Later, he revealed that he was wracking his brain to remember where he'd seen me before. Meanwhile I stared, curious as could be about this suit-and-tie man who wanted to help a bunch of pagans. It was typical of our differences: Kai the disguised and decorous, Sue who barges right in. I knew there was a portent in the air.

Over the next several weeks, his wife proceeded to convince both of us that she was in the throes of converting to lesbianism. Legal matters with Kai turned into chitchat, then more. At gatherings where his wife regaled one and all with her flaming personality, he and I would wind up in a corner staring into one another's eyes.

What *was* responsible for the fire between us? Obviously, we both faced major turning points. When Kai's wife made a definitive play for me, I politely refused, but it signaled the end of an era for him. I was unmarried, and the passion to join with someone who could see beyond my Fringe Woman façade was overwhelming. We understood each other, down to the core.

Renegade yet stable, the maverick that fit in: this was my approving appraisal of Kai Brinkhoff. He managed it, I would later understand, at a cost. But in the beginning it looked as though he'd accomplished a feat that was virtually alchemical, a blending of two worlds into the gold of success. The time had come for me to forsake the so-called sensitive men, the losers and loners full of New Age-speak who were so treacherously absent when the real soul-work of relationships loomed nigh.

So I married a man with a television set, someone who paid for cable and kept its nightly rituals. Who was already married to his career (an oversight easily missed in the delicious months of courtship). A man who loved sports and shopping, had certain obsessive-compulsive traits and heartily ate meat. On the surface, it appeared that I was ripe for rescue from one too many strange rangers.

When two persons have soul-business they must complete, it seems they'll run over anyone in their path. We were guilty as charged, and took our wedding vows in a pagan circle that mentioned past lives and the next one.

But there was more at stake. Two people who'd made it to midlife avoiding parenthood were a set-up for sizable karmic trickery of some magnitude. It didn't take long before we acknowledged the task before us. We had been waiting, seemingly, for each other in order to do this. Birth control was put aside since we agreed we weren't getting any younger.

In retrospect, there is no other explanation: we were, for each other, the one needed to complete the mission. To be shattered and reborn by the experience of parenting, to be aged and made glad, sober, and mad by the unexpected package that was our child.

It would not, however, take place through this womb.

Missed carrying

Four times, a viable fetus failed to make it past the earliest stage. Four times I took to the land, setting spells, praying hard, rolling naked on the breast of Mother Earth. It should have worked, but for the first time ever magic let me down. The Goddess withdrew and withheld.

Searing migraines seemed a mild inconvenience compared to being denied the most mystical experience available to a human being—or so said a number of women who'd given birth. Since we forget our own emergence into gravity and light and arrive too late on the other side to describe our death, pushing a new being from the womb seemed like nirvana for the socially acceptable taking.

Still, I hungered more for the day-to-day of parenting than for those nine months gestating the experience. *Do it, or you'll never know what you need to know.* Once I met Kai, I thought it was all about him; it would complete us.

At least the land was ours and I could have it all to myself, grieving privately and alone after each miscarriage. Kai could not handle the letdowns. His own beloved mother had died shortly after our wedding, and we were making more visits to the fertility doctors. To this day Kai swears he doesn't blame me for the losses, even after his sperm count showed normal and motile enough. But who wouldn't?

The givers

Enter the child who would make us whole. Who would heal the wounds of *infertility, miscarriage,* and *adoption*, plus all the exhaustion they entail.

We didn't know she was coming.

We knew someone was out there, someone trying to make a lasting stay in my womb, yet each time ejected after a mere few weeks. The doctors said I was too old. Meanwhile, everyone had a tale about a first-time Madonna at the age of the big four-zero. I was forty-four years of age when the phone rang with a voice from the past, ready to explode the present beyond all recognition.

"Sue! Is it really you? Sandra Boone here."

Of course I remembered her. Hard-core Osage End hippies, she and her husband had been friends of my lesser friends, who were mostly friends of my ex. We hung out together at parties where any depth of relationship went up in smoke, as it were. When Sandra called that day out of nowhere, she made short work of the pleasantries that a lost acquaintance expects to hear, and came right to the point.

"How's your adoption process going?" she asked. Sandra explained that she knew we were contracted with an agency to adopt a child because, as an ob-gyn nurse, she had the confidences of doctors like ours.

"Dead in the water," I replied.

What had I been doing for the last five years? Giving my body four chances to labor to no end, home studies, background checks, forms and more forms, plus fingerprinting, scraping together the cash for a foreign adoption, losing a baby just assigned because a typhoon hit the village, getting a passport and then getting…no one. Even if I didn't have the stretch marks beneath my clothes, I thought we'd been through enough.

Sandra unveiled her plan. She suggested that tiny infant Nina might come to our home and stay. Forever. It seemed that the Boones' son and his girlfriend needed to give up their new baby, pronto. "Blond hair and blue eyes"—her voice softened—"she's beautiful." Then the anguish poured through: she was giving us first option on her first grandchild, barely eight weeks old.

Sandra and Aidan Boone hailed from an era when a certain crowd in Osage End rented ramshackle farmhouses, tended organic gardens, and raised goats. Everything I wanted to get back to…someday. While Kai didn't know her from any other stranger, nurses always impressed him. She'd been in obstetrics a long time and babies were her thing. Who better to sell you a baby than an expert? And when she wanted to give you her very own granddaughter—how flattering was that?

Sandra explained that after son Zeke and girlfriend Carol had the baby, they realized they couldn't care for her. They were living in their van. They had no money. Carol had another child already. The extra work and expense of this baby girl was not foreseen.

Sandra had been cleaning up her son's messes for a long time. "Just poor and stupid" was how she described the two, assuring us that their problems were neither drug- nor alcohol-related. Zeke was in love, traveling the country, acting as daddy to the little boy—until new baby made one too many.

I couldn't picture Zeke at all. Calling up hazy memories of a cherub toddler, cute and curly, I could hardly believe that Zeke, as new papa, was eighteen years old. His main concern about us, as adoptive parents, was what kind of car did we drive?

Filled in by our physician, Sandra knew the hunger we were dealing with. She said Zeke and Carol could arrive with the baby the next day. It took us a week to get everything ready, and during that time we ventured nightly over to Sandra and Aidan's house to stare blissfully at the one who would topple all my views about nurture-versus-nature.

We knew nothing about babies and loved every weird thing Nina did. We were terrified to hold her at first, and she bristled at this. We watched her sleep, and we watched her commune—with objects.

Staring at bright lights, her whole body shaking as if in paroxysms of joy, wild fists in the air, moved to the core of her tiny self. "How cute." We were awed. Baby antics. Baby mysteries.

The Boones had a parakeet, vocal and shrill. Held up to view the cage, Nina shook from shoulders to wrists, flapping like a fellow bird. "Her arms are her barometer," remarked Sandra. I liked the way she phrased it. The baby expert knew things we didn't.

Then the moment arrived to bring her home. After one last dinner out as a childless couple, we loaded up bassinet, diapers, stroller, and baby blankets. Sandra held her composure, but Aidan looked a wreck. He was always the distant, morose sort—the kind to emerge with a cutting comment, and then close down before you could ponder it. On our nightly visits to watch the baby he stayed in the background, mute. That night I had to block out his face, ravaged with loss. Not that our fireworks of joy could be dampened. Nor could I have envisioned the steps that Aidan would take later—dancing toward, then away.

Kai drove home like an old man at the wheel, careful of our precious cargo. At 2:00 a.m., when the baby woke crying, needing a change, needing a bottle, we welcomed ourselves to the audacity of nights shaped by demand.

The first year was bliss.

Chapter 11
WARRIORS FOR HER CAUSE

There's nothing like having a baby to forget the past.

There I go again: "Before we *had* Nina, since we *had* Nina…" People always cut in with, "I thought you said she was adopted?"

Okay, then, before we *got* Nina. I bow before the need to distinguish biological production from the act of procurement. One is not allowed to actively *have* a child that was produced in another's womb. Never mind that the adoption process is a far harder and longer labor than pregnancy. But the language of acquisition always bugs me, so I opt for "since Nina came into our lives." I figure she picked us, anyway.

There was that thing about karma again. Maybe it creates a stronger, unseen placenta between those who don't happen to hook up in the flesh. I believed it every time I looked into Nina's extraordinary blue eyes. Although she cried and struggled the first time I held her at the Boones' house, I knew it was the *energy* of my nervousness that upset her. Never, at that moment, did I feel she hated me, or that it would be a long haul to her heart. From the beginning Nina was like that: assertive. *If you can't calm the hell down, let go of me!* That was the imperative message of her wordless, two-month-old cries as Sandra and Aidan looked on, drawing who knows what conclusions.

Stepping into Babyland isn't just a rite of passage, it's a gateway to the all-consuming Now. I never ceased reminding The Judge of the irony.

"You said I wasn't thinking about my future? Copping out with some blather about the eternal present? Well, Your Honor, how's poop, spit, vomit, and unsound sleep for a future filled with Now?"

Even without milk in the breasts or a uterus to recover, a parent can be fully equipped with radar and love. Receiving grandparents and friends in the days following Nina's arrival, I was often told, "You look so proud," with an accusatory twinkle.

"I'm proud of her, can't you see how beautiful she is? I'm just happy. Ecstatic, in fact."

Nina was a hard-won prize. We were proud to have her on board. We were so proud of her that we passed off every strange thing she did for far too long. We thought of it as the kid simply being herself—or perhaps not herself, *today*.

✳ ✳ ✳

Nina's laughing at the ceiling again.

A squat pillar of baby fat, steady on her new feet for once, eyes glued to her favorite corner of the screened porch where cedar meets pine. Kai and I look up, too. Maybe this time we'll get the joke. Or see the apparition. But the ceiling looks bare, with not even a bumbling bug trying to find its way out. No hanging plant or outdoor do-dad dangling—there is nothing but air, and whatever it is Nina alone can see.

Goaded to mirth, she forgets us. She only has eyes for whatever, whoever, is on the ceiling—and the conversation looks juicy.

"Didn't know dead people were so funny." Kai knows just what I mean.

After we bought the house, stories seeped in of former occupants who had "seen things" in mirrors, in the hallway, on the hill out back. The numerous pottery shards and arrowheads found in the yard and nearby creek twisted anthropology into ooga-booga. We believed it and yet we didn't, fixated on something even more miraculous: the first baby for either of us, both past forty and counting. Still, after one year in the house, Nina laughed at things neither of us could see.

"Awwwwww." She bends over, unleashing a fresh load of giggles. Jealous of the competition, we try to win her back with a word, a tickle, a toy. She struggles to stay intent on the ceiling, on the ghost.

It is her gift, we believe, to frequent other planes. With envy and awe, we watch her fascination with the inconspicuous. In the backyard she thrills to leaf, wind, and smooth bark as they conspire in a shrub that captivates her. The fronds sway, then stop—nothing special, but she hovers for the greater part of an hour, hands waving at their stillness or sudden movements, nose so close to a faded flower that those beautiful blue eyes cross.

"She sees fairies," I whisper. "Our Nina's going to be a mystic—probably a healer."

Then came the morning when I faced the fact that she had spent an hour curled up and tapping on a wall, with the saddest look I'd ever seen on a toddler's face. It was starting to happen a lot.

Couch potato-esque, we called her. She sat. It didn't matter—we loved holding her, sweeping her up in our arms to get her from one place to the next. No longer did she crave whirling in a circular motion without getting dizzy, a move we called "dancing." Nor was she interested in being outdoors. She never said a word.

Among other things, I'd seen motherhood as another building block in my immunity against the Wohler Madness. I'd sensibly waited until I was older, married to my soul mate, surrounded by beautiful acres of woods and prairie. Yet it came to pass that the Wohler Madness came stalking me at last. Not with voices and visions, addictions or mania, but with unlifting dread and anxiety as I tried my hardest to do the right thing for a daughter I couldn't understand.

Opening the door to experts

After that initial year of bliss, we waited for our daughter's first word: "Daddy!" It happened once, never to be heard again. We talked and talked to her, we read, we whooped, we bombarded her with sensible nouns. How easily one overlooked what was missing: a look straight in the eye, a cuddle leaned into like it was second nature to bond. We made excuses, or entertained the thought that she didn't love us at all.

Well into her second year, Nina remained listless before her toys. She sat beside the bottled water fixture with her tiny nails flicking the spigot, not thirsty. She piled toys on top of furniture in precarious towers, and then set out to climb them. She ran into walls, and felt not a thing. She booby-trapped our sleep with wrenching screams into the night. *Something's wrong.*

At age two, mute and inactive, Nina was stalled. Kai and I agreed: a little speech therapy, that's all she needs! The professionals were called. They came and they stayed for their little half hour, once or twice a week, while I ached at the closed door—and after they left Nina was still not *here*.

Medical doctors said she was fine.

How the A-word moved in, like a relative who never meant to stay so long, I can't recall. The therapists, so careful not to alarm us, never spoke it. As if the word itself invoked the devil, as if we'd take holy offense. As if, Goddess forbid, she might be One of Those. *Autism,* that word, meant the end of the world.

So we agreed to the fancy evaluation in Kansas City.

❊ ❊ ❊

Two weeks and counting: we will soon take Nina in to see if the dreaded diagnosis fits.

Kai walks into the room. "You know they're going to find her autistic," he says, scrutinizing my face for cracks. I'm shocked; I thought he was in on the going-through-the-motions, let's-humor-the-Special Educators with me. "Probably high-functioning," he adds when he sees me blanch, as if that's a consolation. And it is—a scrap of something saved. We won't completely hit bottom.

I have some time to read up on this thing that Nina is *(please, please)* not. So I head to the temple, the Science Library, located in the same complex where Nina's judges await her.

Call numbers steer me from the Liberal Arts repository, that venerable dark edifice down the road where my kind hunches in stacks not quite lit, not quite clean. By contrast, the Science Library is a cathedral, full of light and inlaid stone. The quiet isn't close, it ambles and soars. There's no ostentation, though, just everything I need to know about the psyche, from schizophrenia to the impact of sexual abuse to upbeat topics like autism. Here I come to fill my mind like a sail.

But first: this is where my ancestor is kept alive. Into the terminal I type his name: *Wohler, Friedrich.*

There he is, or rather his works—on minerals, meteorites, and medicine, in both English and German. I've been told he is family but somehow, sitting here, I feel I'm sharing him with everyone who walks by. He probably never heard the word *autism,* never met an autistic person. Never even sensed, I'll wager, the epidemic ahead.

Autism beats out Wohler for the number of entries on-line, and I surf for a place to land: *The Riddle of Autism: A Psychological Analysis*, by George Victor. Of course I'm drawn to this one: whatever ails our Nina, surely, is trauma carried from the womb she stormed despite an IUD, plus those first few weeks of living with the "poor and stupid" birth parents in their car.

Dr. Victor does his best to unpack the causes of autism, formerly heaped upon cold-hearted, intellectual parents. He grants that the charge of "refrigerator mothers" was unfair, so at first I'm with him. Autism, he asserts, is a bona fide developmental disability, not the result of mean, icy moms. Then he veers into history: in rural Europe, all psychotic and retarded offspring were once called "children of God." In Ireland, well into the mid-twentieth century, their births were thought to be a blessing on the mother and a good omen for the community.

I knew it! Nina is an old soul.

Dr. Victor then explains that parents of autistic children labor under the delusion of a child "destined for greatness." Their fantasizing begins before birth, he posits, with assertions of an "extraordinary conception." He pleads with readers to see how it's all "part of the myth of the coming of the hero."

On it goes, steadily downhill. The parents are "infatuated" with such children. Consequently, autism produces "the sensual child," a highly autoerotic creature, a being who is "superstitious…inscrutable." When not masturbating the day away, these children *self-induce* an epileptic seizure to *enjoy* the stimulation. Their chronic gastrointestinal problems are a product of "stress" due to "negativism on the part of the parents." (You heard that right: infatuated, but negative.) "Perhaps the food selectivity of autistic children is regressive attachment behavior with the function of care given young infants."

So that's it—I loved Nina too much. It made her sick. Thank you, Dr. Victor.

✳ ✳ ✳

In our culture, we don't say *womb* very often. Ovaries, clitoris, vulva, the fallopian two—we talk around the womb. It's another w-word, maybe not as prickly as *witch* but just as archaic. As for uterus, the clinical sounds fine when a hysterectomy's at hand. Patriarchy avoids the woo-word as too mysterious (or maybe too mystical?) to describe our first home, that vessel of our maiden voyage.

A woman senses the womb's weight when blood drops on a lunar rhythm, or when she cramps with that effort. We are not aware of a cavern, of a space making ready for passengers; we look at diagrams and feel as alienated as the next woman about our "plumbing." I didn't block the possibilities of a womb from mind before my marriage to Kai because it was yucky—I was simply afraid of being trapped.

Raised in the 1950's, I had to confront my mother's life, that cordoning off of women from the world of work, politics, sports, money. Barefoot and pregnant: a suburban form of indentured servitude equaled *womb*. Tied to a man and beholden to his domain, what if the man turned out to be Caligula? There you were—stuck.

Visions of the dependency that pregnancy and birth entailed were flipped on end by the wild Goddess, who seemed anything but weak in her birth-giving. But the ticking of the biological clock also transformed many an inchoate resistance. I found myself ready to embark, not so much for the body trip, but to get inside the mystery, maybe rub shoulders with the Great Mother I'd been tracking all this time.

The gloomy aftermath of each miscarriage was deepened by Kai's anger and distance. I went to the creek where sitting stones welcomed in a crook of its meander, the water making a change of heart right before it ran into a hill. There I sang my sorrow. With life renewing itself all around me in the seasonal round, I prayed for a better next-time. I'd never been told "no" before by the Earth, so I invited the spirits of missed babies to come to the oak trees, to bask on the stones, play in the creek. I still had faith.

After the fourth miscarriage, faith was wracked by persistent tremors. Through the Goddess I'd finally embraced the womb, but missed the chance to carry anyone there. I lost babies in winter and honored the tie-in to loss and death, knowing that such experiences were part of the Crone, the eldest of the Goddess' triple aspect. Because I kept hearing the same old excuses about my age and infertility, I beseeched the Crone to prove the doctors wrong.

Nina's coming meant I was back in Her good graces—the Goddess had meant *this* instead. Those beautiful blue, utterly observant eyes, before the turn to sadness. How *could* she be so bereft, when we lived and died for every moment we shared with her? When the land all around her, all hers, greened and waved and said, *Run to me, you are mine!*

I often put Nina on my lap while I sat on the creek's biggest stone, flat and broad as if made for a chair, and surrounded by flow. I didn't come for "parts parties" anymore—no psychic parts needed to duke it out, hammer an agreement. There were no issues. Kai was a daddy, charmed and involved, Nina was beauty incarnate, and I was on the parenting high.

But as I looked down the barrel of an autism diagnosis, I didn't know what to make of Her design. I didn't really believe in fate, in a Goddess who decrees and decides. I'd spent so long figuring out that I was always and forever aligned with Her will. Then She tricked me, offered me a whole year that felt like life was back on track, only to follow it with this bomb: *the baby wasn't right.*

Was I really so shallow that my "spiritual connectedness" rose and fell with my happiness over how daily life turned out?

The Goddess could probably care less whether I was having a good day, or a miscarriage. I wanted to keep some rational wits about me, not pout as if She were a parent who'd been withholding, testing my loyalty. If this was a test, I reasoned, I had brought it on myself by shedding my Fringe Woman persona, by taking chances on some middle-class concept of marriage. I would mine the ordeal for meaning, sure. But I could not bring myself to talk to the Moon.

And I'd never seen anything like autism in nature, either. Autism was not natural. Then what was Nina?

Lost connections

The grandparent Boones originally thought they wanted to be involved in Nina's life, but nurse Sandra couldn't handle it. It's not exactly that she couldn't take the adoption. She couldn't handle any alteration to her fantasy that we would assimilate into *their* family, and she would remain the grand dame at the center of it all.

I gently asked for a little time to ourselves after we'd brought Nina home. I asked again that she please stop saying how much Nina looked like members of their family. I tried to visit as required, but there were uncomfortable incidents. When Sandra held Nina, she and Aidan's seven-year-old child ran from the room crying, "You love *her* more than me!"

Sandra clung to baby Nina and gazed upon her as if transfixed. She alluded constantly to her grief at their parting. Much later, I wondered if her behaviors were rooted in guilt. Kai and I were so ecstatic to finally be a family with a child that we couldn't help her. We supported Sandra in getting professional counseling. Eventually, the grand dame decided that if she couldn't rule, she would not be seen. With great finality, Sandra Boone withdrew.

Yet her husband Aidan stayed. Like someone shedding a cocoon, he came into his own once he was released from his wife's shadow.

Aidan drove out to the woods for a visit, and we were glad to get to know him. He was transformed from the cardboard figure he'd played during the adoption ordeal. Lighting a candle to signal ceremonial space, he claimed Nina as his granddaughter and himself as "Granddaddy." We were grateful for him and envisioned being friends for life.

Aidan embodied the kernel of good that I cherished from my own past. I recalled his passionate involvement in Vietnam Veterans Against the War. After the war, he worked as an advocate for the underdog in his career. Beneath the outer trappings, he told us, he was unchanged from his sixties values and convictions.

Maybe he was the wrong person to tell when I realized Nina didn't do what other children her age did. Still, I needed someone to talk to. I counted on him—and when we were thinking of having her evaluated, I needed to know his thoughts.

"She doesn't have autism," he said flat out. We were on the front porch where Nina loved to look up at the ceiling and laugh.

"I agree. At least, I want to."

"What's the pediatrician say?"

"She says, 'Her? Autistic? I don't think so.'"

"Well, there you have it."

"Yeah, but I'm not so sure the family practitioners are up on this."

"I don't see it. She responds when I talk to her." Aidan glanced over at Nina, sitting dazed on the piano bench, her back to the keys.

"I get that. She's a loving child, or at least she was before this change. But why isn't she talking to us?"

"All kinds of kids are late talkers. Zeke needed speech therapy in the fourth grade, some consonants and stuff he couldn't quite spit out right."

"And what about his, uh, troubled adolescence? Tell me more."

"We took him to this place and that place, but they could never figure out what was wrong with him. He just hated school. We'd drop him off at the front door and he'd walk right out the back. He was into cars."

"Oh, like my little brother."

"No, I mean like hot-wiring one now and then for a joy ride."

"Yikes. But Carol, the birth mom...is there anything else you haven't told me?"

Sandra had made it clear that Zeke's choice of girlfriend was not what she'd hoped for her son. Carol had been raised by one of Osage End's chronically homeless families. They'd lived in their car. Before Zeke, Carol had had a son by a former husband. Zeke was involved heart and soul in parenting the little boy.

Aidan knew where I was trying to take this. I'd asked before if drugs and alcohol had been part of the birth parents' life. Fetal alcohol syndrome would explain a lot of Nina's problems. But Sandra swore to the negative. I remembered once again her twin adjectives for the pair: poor and stupid.

Now Aidan was without his wife's opinion to hide behind.

"I've never seen them even take a drink. With all the substances I consumed way back when, I can tell when someone's hiding something. Frankly, it's like they're too young. I mean, they're old enough to drink, but they're like little kids in grown-up bodies playing house—when they have a house. They like to go to Wal-Mart; they like to ride in their van. I've told you about the half-dozen jobs they've been through in just two years." Aidan sighed. "Don't ask me to figure out my son. I try not to think about it."

I needed Aidan's support and Kai did, too. Without Sandra's over-bearing presence, we looked forward to Aidan whenever we saw his white pickup nosing up the driveway. He was talkative, generous, and devoted to Nina to the very end. This, apparently for him, came when her diagnosis was confirmed.

D-Day

Nina thrashed in my arms, a thirty-two-pound rocket ready to take off as the doctor walked ahead of us. My daughter's blonde pageboy was matted on a face turning scarlet, her screams readable enough. She was fed up with this maze.

I hadn't explained this place ahead of time, much less the need to stay. Neither the concept of "doctor" nor a sneaky "Let's go play!" was hers to grasp, so I'd highlighted the car ride, a favorite pastime. Except for oddly pitched yelps and bleeps, Nina said little in return. The famous blue eyes remained downcast, just like they did on most days now.

Diaper bag slung over an aching shoulder, raingear stuffed into an armpit, and girl writhing on my hip, I moved like a slow barge into the next little room. Nina was no infant, and strangers frequently mis-took me for her grandmother. She often chose to ride in a parent's arms, so scared was she of anywhere new. I was beginning to think she could read the vibe of a place, and this one was portentous.

Kai handed over the stack of forms that we'd finally completed. The door closed. Dad checked Nina's diaper, hoping to avoid another of those exploding poops. The three of us were told to wait, and we did as we were told.

We'd just seen a medical doctor in a white coat who had specu-lated about "Fragile X," the little chromosome that could explain every out-of-kilter thing about Nina. But that genetic fault wasn't common, and it was obvious that she was just making conversation to pass the time before the verdict: a thumbs-up, or else the A-word for life.

It was D-Day: Diagnosis Day.

So far the ordeal had consisted of shuttling from one cubicle to the next, where yet another professional held out a satchel of toys de-signed to reveal The Truth about child development. At the moment, however, there was no plan apparent. I eased Nina, still clueless in the third year of her life, onto the cushioned exam table and checked the backs of my hands for scratches. She had a way of taking things out on others.

Nina promptly hid her eyes from the bright fluorescents overhead as Kai and I took a breather. No toys, no charts on the wall. No explanation about how long the wait, or why. Yet there was one unique feature that marked this stop: a single mirror in which we could gaze at our harried selves. Its silver expanse was half a wall wide, and stretched long and gleaming without a smudge.

Kai frowned and approached the glass. "Look at this," he said, "the thing's transparent."

Nina was face down, fetal, curled up to stay. I joined him and stood against the wall, unable to penetrate the mirror's face. But he knew how to look.

"It's a two-way," he said. "People are on the other side, pulling up chairs."

I groaned under the weight of this last straw and went back to my crumpled-up kid. The mirror was a window! "They" would be watching! And what if they saw us watching them? Would our knowing that we were being spied on be misinterpreted by the spies?

And what if, somehow, that blew it for our daughter? By now, surely, our judges were taking notes while we stood stumped. What should we make her do for them?

What the evaluators didn't know was that Kai was once the youngest city administrator in the country. At age twenty, in a small town in western Kansas, he had purchased two-way mirrors for the diminutive police department. Thus, a mix of indignity and gall provoked my husband to keep himself pressed against the wall next to the shiny thing for a peek. They were still there, the folks testing Nina, each with their special expertise in the diagnostic category we dreaded to take home.

Autism.

That day, we learned they test parents too.

Kai finally sat down and we defaulted to silence, patting the immobile Nina. We forced some chitchat about the unusual August downpour, stealing glances at the mirror. I tried to interest Nina in a picture book fetched from her bag, unsure of how a perfect mom should do this, until I could stand it no longer.

"What now?" I whispered. "This is too weird! It's 1999—I thought they didn't believe parents caused autism anymore. Do you think they're listening?"

"Oh, I think so," Kai answered in his large-lungs way, and stood up.

Don't do it! I thought, and then, *too late, they'll hear me, and write who knows what about the spousal dynamic.* But I knew the man enough to know when he was on a mission. Resigned to whatever came next (and I knew it wouldn't be good), I watched Kai stride over to a light sconce near the mirror and start feeling around the base. Finding at last what he was looking for, his smirk spoke volumes, but naturally he had to say it out loud.

"May they listen well!"

Tapping hard on the hidden microphone with an extended, deliberate rat-a-tat, Nina's dad glared through the looking glass, bucking for a label of his own.

Fascinated onlookers

After all the tests, the chill in the judgment room was palpable. Am I making this up, or was the air-conditioner cranked to maximum? A whole row of staff sitting at a table like panelists, facing us like one solid iceberg. Did this have anything to do with Kai blowing out their eardrums in the peeping room?

There was a practiced quality to their restraint; they used the fewest words possible and kept faces of stone. They were curious about us. We were a phenomenon: parents on the edge of a diagnosis that was gaining in application these days, with no certain cause. What interesting data might we present in our reaction?

Barely a muscle or sheet of paper moved until the chief clinician produced a telling graph that showed Nina's score, placing her clearly in the spectrum that is designated autism. I left Kai to hear the rest of it and fled the room. Nina was in my arms, oblivious to my tears as I squeezed her, sobbed on her, rocked her for every and no reason.

What was this thing, autism? Not quite the Wohler Madness, which I could deny with all of my theories stacked and polished to a tee. Not political repression, for which collective activism was the cure. Not even gender-specific—in fact, it favored boys four to one. It fit no known category of description or solution.

Sitting on the thin, worn cushions of the waiting room while Kai endured the iceberg, I invoked the Amazon within and without. To be a warrior for her cause—there was no hesitation, because Nina was me. I had been thrown away as a child, once I began to see past Clark Gable to the real Narcissus who was my dad. I was the black sheep, the bad seed, the next in line to receive the enduring mantle of the family disease. My Inner Child was healed, but she still begged for my loyalty. She was the most enthusiastic champion Nina had.

I remembered the Habitat. I would never, ever abandon Nina. There was no question of whether I was going to step up and take care of this child. My fate-date with Kai demanded it; many other reasons to stand by her would be patched in later, horrors I didn't go looking to discover. All I knew, at that moment, was what I'd heard and read and everyone agreed: despite the ever-unfolding palette of new treatments, there was still no cure.

No cure.

Why ditch me, Goddess of my heart?

I soon realized that people who knew me were acting like they didn't.

I hadn't noticed life going on while I read about autism, studied Nina in a new light, made therapy appointments, and tried to face the A-word head on so as to nip its bulbous bud as soon as possible. This was a battle—why weren't more of my friends in the trenches besides me?

For one thing, autism was all I could talk about. My grief pushed past any stopper. Sympathy was there for the taking, but only once or twice per person. Then, apparently, it was time to move on. How do you heal from such a loss when a person's not dead—but not really here, either?

Second, if the Goddess stiffed me in terms of a biological child, then this was some further cruel joke on Her part. Should I do another ritual? For what? A miracle cure, when all agreed there was no cure? I expected results from magic, or at least a cessation of pain. I dropped all pretenses of faith and outright blamed Her.

Third, it had been a while since we had been able to take Nina anywhere in public. She stood out as clearly not up to the level of other toddlers. She was tired. She had nothing to say and took no interest in others. Sounds bothered her and strange places were a jumble of sights. We didn't want to make her life harder. But we didn't know who we were anymore, either.

What could "earth-based spirituality" do? What relevance did it have now? I hovered on the verge of a bitterness that scared the daylights out of me. So I just fought harder. Because the Goddess gave me the Amazons to emulate and because, despite always being set one step aside from "real" or biological mothers, I was Nina's mom. At least Rebel Girl had taught me a few tricks. Nina needed every ally within me. Who else did she have?

Distant men

After D-Day, Kai's attitude and approach to Nina changed. The shift was abrupt, final, puzzling. She had been his world. "You may be Queen Mother," he laughed, pointing at me, "but she is The Queen." I thought nothing could break their bond. Did he feel pushed aside by the momentum of my warrior fire as it came onboard for her?

But Aidan was the male figure who literally cut out on Nina, never calling us to discuss her diagnosis—or anything else, ever again. Others left just by changing their attitudes toward her. For Kai, the cooling off was immediate. I didn't understand how he could be so glued to his profession, fighting the good fight for the oppressed (many of his legal clients were disabled) and yet *not* throw himself into a quest for her quality of life. I never understood why he wouldn't stand beside me as a fellow warrior, for the Amazons were known to consort with sympathetic men.

To be fair, he did put nose to the grindstone even harder to meet the financial challenges. They were mounting and we couldn't keep up. We knew we weren't doing the *crème-de-la-crème* treatments—they were too high-dollar. Kai did interface with the school district whenever needed; after all, there was something about having a man, a persuasive attorney, grousing at them that seemed to prod them to try harder.

Research suggests that fear of inadequacy is a major cause of men's indifference to their special needs children. Perhaps the urge in Kai to give Nina everything was so strong, yet met so painfully by limitation, that he couldn't deal with it. So he shut down. He left the house to find his kudos from people who knew nothing about her.

My father, now recovered from a triple bypass and fit as a fiddle, also changed toward Nina. No big surprise there. We were disappointing him, Benny and I, giving him grandkids who would have no chance of being smarter than the average bear. Ben and his wife had adopted two half-brothers from Cambodia who turned out to have "problems." By preschool the label *attention deficit hyperactivity disorder* had been draped around them, and they were off to a special school.

When I first made Robert and Marie Elton grandparents, Nina's arrival seemed to turn the tide so that whatever happened in that little mental hospital on the prairie was entirely forgiven. Benny had already provided them with the opportunity to learn the ropes of grandparenting, and when I finally got on the bandwagon my parents strolled into my life as if we were in a new world. I was willing: I had better things to focus on than their crimes. I thought it would be good for my kid to have grandparents. I also had a lever: Nina was mine, so let them misbehave and *you know what.* No more Nina in their lives.

Since she was the first girl of the bunch, they doted on her in ways that were new to the game for them. We all ate it up. I didn't feel so much that I was finally accepted or that they were particularly off the hook, just that it didn't matter anymore. Here was their chance to show me they could do better.

But anything resembling the Wohler Madness proved to be too much for them to take. Add in the need for remedial education, and my father took it as a minor scandal. Narcissus lost his chip off the old block to brag about. D-Day was the end of an era, short but concilia-tory, between my father and me.

✳ ✳ ✳

Sam's fate (transferred out of the home and into the hands of a routine residential placement) could have befallen Nina. Every parent of an adult autistic I've met tells that they were advised by profession-als to institutionalize when the child was young. Not that long ago, autism and schizophrenia were considered synonymous. But for once I was in the right place at the right time.

In 1964, a brave parent-researcher named Dr. Bernard Rimland refused to accept the psychological theories of the day that blamed distant, cold parents for turning a child far, far inward. He refuted the work of psychologist Bruno Bettelheim, a Freudian who had reinforced the notion of "refrigerator mothers," as he and his wife searched for a way to help their autistic child.

Bernard Rimland had to dig deep, translate obscure German articles, and piece together the puzzle in a novel way, but with time came the answer. Autism is a neurological condition, not the deliber-ate response of a perfectly normal mind that chooses mute retreat. It was neither madness nor retardation, but their more mysterious twin. Born with the condition or developing before the age of five, autistic minds were wired very differently from the neurotypical, resulting in idiosyncratic patterns or pure deficits in speech and social interaction.

This was very big news, but it would take decades for any finger to point in the direction of a real, physiological cause.

I organized my psyche's life around this one truth: *she's not crazy.* Nina's problem was developmental, not mental. She was not blood-related—the Wohler Madness could not touch her. I suppose I blamed the birth parents for not gifting Nina with a great start in life, although that was hard to dwell on considering they graciously made us par-ents, too. At the time I wanted to believe that autism just happens, but I couldn't erase the thought that kept running on an endless tape: *if she had been born of my womb….*

But she wasn't.

Surely this was the Goddess' last prank—how could She top it? I guessed we could all die in a fire or a car wreck. But then we'd be on the Other Side and Nina could talk, tell us she loved us, and Kai wouldn't have to work so hard.

Chapter 12
THE OPIATES OF THE PEOPLE

Mr. Normal is on the job.

By daylight Kai drinks coffee and then charges forth, a practice that reeks of adulthood. I watch him sip and hunker down to business like someone who can forget there is an autistic child in the house. He does normal on very little shut-eye. "Sleeping," he pronounces, "is a waste of time."

Sleep, of course, was one place the Wohler Madness could never get me in the decades before Nina. The dream journals! The down comforters! Best of all, still lying around at noon. "Your thing about sleep," Kai scoffs, "is truly a fetish."

We step around the hardest fact of all: after nine years of parenting without sleep, there is little rest in sight. Nina does not go gentle into her good night.

The rare full night's rest comes like a single bite to a starving inmate, a taste that will not be repeated soon. My dreams are of endless journeys navigating crowded cities, missing deadlines, losing my tickets or a map. That's all I can recall after waking repeatedly to the sound of Nina's distress.

Red numbers on the digital clock burn. A robe wraps and unwraps all night long. Slow bones take to the floor while trying to sequence what comes next.

Darkening her door with a bottle, staying longer, touching her, trying not to get mad or cry along, deeply sorry for myself. When infancy gave way to a bigger kid who still punctuated the night with her demands, those minutes in Nina's room weighed hard. Kai watched TV and waited for his turn to minister to our daughter. Or he slept ahead in twisted sheets: the breadwinner, taking his too-short hours of wasted time.

At first we told ourselves to get used to it. All children periodically need something in the night. Comes with the territory.

Maybe. But every single night, with screams? *These* screams? Does every parent hear these same inconsolable, mystery screams? The first notes blast full force, a cry of "lost in the wilderness." Then the steady voice of Nina's pain: neither real rage, nor real calling, merely indecipherable.

I had a solution that she sought every two or three hours—a silicon nipple, given without shame. Thankfully, every bout of screams was finally quelled by milk. If I couldn't give her the breast, at least the calcium that builds strong bones. Vicariously my body dispensed, hand on bottle, as if it were part of my flesh.

Betrayed by food

Two weeks after D-Day, Kai and I sat among our brethren and told ourselves we weren't like them. They looked strained and bedraggled, these parents of autistic children. We studied the small, blond, business-like woman setting up at the front of the room; she promised answers. A parent-researcher with an autistic son, she was about to divulge what others had not.

At least she had information to offer when I called her, having garnered her name from the iceberg in Kansas City. Most of the others on the list had children grown and gone to group homes. They couldn't really help us, and seemed surprised that the clinic still gave out their names. They were a beaten-down lot, with little hope to trade.

Betty Bolen was different. Her modus was precision, science, documentation. Her heart was set to give hope—not the syrupy kind, but hard-nosed evidence. It all boiled down to three startling things that she told us:

1. Milk from cows is a drug to our kids.

2. Wheat (or *gluten*, also found in barley, rye, and other grains) acts in the same way. When ingested, both dairy products and gluten made for altered states in our children and thus the outward signs of autism.

3. There are micro-beasts in the stomachs of our kids that most mainstream doctors refuse to believe in, a yeast called *candida albicans* that was populating out of control and magnifying autistic symptoms.

Betty Bolen stood up to tell us that autism could be cured by going gluten-free, dairy-free, and attacking those yeast beasts with all our might.

Milk, grower of children, food that stands on its own, the moustache on celebrity billboards. Got milk? Who would have suspected it might be an enemy, perhaps for more of us than are willing be counted? It was all so molecular and abstract. The chemistry was beyond me, still stuck at the level of the Four Major Food Groups.

Neither Kai nor I had heard of this vicious cycle of comfort and assault hidden so innocently in the udders of sweet-eyed cows. It was hard to admit that our gourmet cheese could be a ticking time bomb. Wasn't yogurt supposed to help out in the gut? The whole thing sounded a little un-American at first.

"Lactose intolerance" was a picnic compared to this, a mere bellyache next to behavior disorders. Nina was nearly three years old before we heard from Betty Bolen that the guilty party was casein, milk protein—a far more sticky wicket than lactose, the sugar. In the vulnerable, casein can leak through the gut wall into the bloodstream where dairy's by-products do not belong. The brain reads them as a sedative, addictive as opium. After a bottle and some sleep, Nina woke up in the wee hours because she was no longer stoned. She would cry for a bottle first thing.

Sandra Boone had told us that Nina's half-brother had a milk allergy and drank soy formula. Nina followed suit until our General Practitioner scoffed, and ordered us to get with the cow. So every night I handed over the warmed milk and wondered what was wrong. My child would not come to my lap nor soothe in the nearby rocker. She lived for milk sucked down while flat on her back, same as in daylight. At least on the floor I could lay beside her (without cuddling, of course). Although she appeared to enjoy affection at other moments, her relationship with Bottle was sacred. We'd ponder the blank ceiling together; I'd mosey in as close as I could, holding the milky cylinder that eased her pain. Her eyes slid sideways in my direction, but for the most part she communed with the spirits of casein and waited for her hit to take effect.

Where was the Nina who should have been brandishing a bottle upright, with nipple clamped in tiny teeth? I studied the dexterity of other babies who twirled their milk batons in public. But Nina couldn't hold the thing herself. I perched on a stool, leaning over the crib rail to hold the vessel for her and told myself, *Surely she's not picking up on how weird I am. She's not pulling away because of me, not me in particular.*

But what do I do for her? I did nothing, while Nina surrendered to the cascade of opiates beguiling the neurons they would target next. Such was my baby's drug of choice.

Trounced

In no time I quit socializing altogether. Like my grandmother, I tried to cope with a family—and loneliness. Like my paranoid brother, I felt myself cast adrift into a world where I had nothing in common with anyone. Having a child with autism set me apart, though that was a secondary concern. What the disorder was doing to this child entrusted to me to raise was the hardest part to bear. The toll taken when you must attend to such a young being's suffering daily, not really knowing what to do.

Kai dealt with his grief over Nina's diagnosis by nit-picking everything I said and did. There was no time for magic, for the creek, for a sunset. My life as a wild woman and priestess of the Earth seemed like a book I read long ago. I Can Do This became my daily mantra amidst the enclosure of home, as I lusted for uninterrupted sleep in a wide bed alone. But after the baby-high wore into toddler-grind, I admitted I was slipping.

How could I end up as one of those depressed mothers? I'd had it all planned: after some full-time parenting, a careful step back into my career as the village witch. But familiarity with my own plans was fading. I had let my clients go, one by one, during the infertility-and-adoption years. Now finally a parent, I was more confused by my child than I'd ever been by a client—how could I help anyone now? I measured my moxie by the fact I could still bitch loudly and pray fervently for more stamina. Until finally, inevitably, stopped in my tracks, I would fold into the revenge of the migraines, more ferocious than ever.

Wincing at lights and shrill child babble, my focus was only on getting through. Bottoming out came two to three times per week as Nina showed no signs of sleeping through the night. There wasn't the option of letting her "cry it out," and besides, it was too easy to hear the meanie inside my head: *You failure, are you still foisting yourself on these people? You think you are a mother; you think this is a family? Imposter!* I'd rather stay moving and tracking Nina's screams than listen to that.

Because being an Amazon for her cause felt like the antithesis of the Wohler Madness, because I felt superior to the housewife-careers of my mother and grandmother, because autism was a bona fide crisis mode, I couldn't accept the gender analysis of what was happening. Clearly Kai could earn more money, so it fell to me to take the helm of this problem—yes, *that* was the stuff of gender wars. But if I'd had his earning power, would it have been the luck of the draw or me on the frontlines, regardless? There were lots of dads on the research and treatment quest, but could Kai have handled it?

I dwelt on another thing. As with Samuel, I couldn't see the Laing-like visionary potential in my daughter's experience. She was glum, she was in pain. Nina was stoned on foods that bopped her brain, reeling from a problem that seemed to be gut-centered. I was learning about the enteric nervous system, the so-called second nervous system of the intestines.

We don't want to think that the brain belongs to the body.

We worship all parts of that matter—gray, disembodied, and supposedly wise—running the show over dumb flesh and slimy innards. Complex and righteous, the lofty brain lords it over the busy gut, the site of most neurotransmitter action in the whole human being—but don't tell the brain that. Don't involve the chugging organs, those miles of intestines pulverizing your gourmet dinner, with the lofty realms of emotion and thought, the birthright to behave as we will ourselves to behave. *Don't make me think about what's Down There.*

I felt profoundly trapped; the more the walls closed in, the less mystical potential presented itself in daily life. Maybe I'd been wrong about all I had been. I no longer wore a pentacle on a silver chain and gave up the flowing long skirts. Such was not the fault of motherhood but the inevitable product of disillusionment.

"You wanted to be a mommy," quipped our plumber-electrician, back one day to repair another breach in the hull of our old house. Friends prescribed more coffee, or commiserated if they were mothers of small children themselves. The TV news told of terrorists' use of sleep deprivation on their hostages. Since I had wanted to be a mommy, I tried to believe that it was natural to feel taken hostage. Yet I'd never seen a baby this old who couldn't hold her own bottle.

Where was Os? I could never relax deeply enough to meet him. It always seemed I was making him up, as opposed to a real presence felt. He looked sheepish at having no answers, no comfort to give. My Inner Child was subsumed into Nina, or in hiding, perhaps, somewhere with Os.

I met each migraine by pouring myself a big glass of milk from the carton stored next to Nina's rice milk in the fridge. Then on to hunks of cheese when the energy dipped so low I could only grab what was at hand. Cheese was love; I reveled in its many textures and tastes. Especially on thick bread, wholly wheat, preferably homemade.

Oh holy head

I started questioning what was going on in my own head when the knell of migraine sounded once too often.

We assume the brain reigns on high, alone and untouched by such baser things as food. To admit its dialogue with the mechanisms of the gut is to dismantle its glorified mystery. The head is where we carry our precious smarts or crazy voices, the hovering head not really connected. Seen in this light, migraines are but the head's simple tendency to dilate its vascular net a tad too wide—but why?

If we allow that some foods are worthy of the brain, then how could stalwart dairy have been a hoax? How I hated to hate the cow! Hadn't I traveled dirt roads through the Flint Hills for fresh-from-the-teat raw milk, hadn't I made my own cheese in a rennet-soaked mass dripping from soft cloth? Just when I wanted to be an exemplary prairie woman, reveling on my own beloved acres, treason called again.

Now when I drove by those innocent four-leggeds, munching contentedly to their death, the bowed heads gave me pause. So many had been my friends on the Finley farm, the dairy cows especially, giving kids rides on their bony backs. I wondered why it took until puberty for their delicious fresh offerings to start giving me screaming headaches. I wondered what might have been different if I'd never tasted a drop of what they had to give. No milk, no Habitat?

The cell we inhabit

Trapped in a house just like my mother, when supposedly there's no need for it nowadays—it wasn't what I expected. Supposedly in this century such a choice is freely chosen and, for some, fulfillment. I craved such intense focus for a year or three, and tolerance for older moms was a trend. I realized that Nina would be my full-time job just when it was time to get back to my life.

Sure, there was the battle aspect to buoy me: draw a sword and defend your own. But who were the villains here? "Disorder" took on a whole new meaning—it was more than what Nina *had*, it was a way of daily life. The chaos of an unpredictable child in clear distress pushes one to search for causation.

Nina had become an unhappy person, fresh out of wisdom, no longer laughing at the ceiling. If she was the Goddess' child, I couldn't fathom the divine plan.

What would Wohler do? I was drawn into that mindset where the science of the body takes precedence over mystical musings. Texts on the brain and behaviorism replaced magical studies on my nightstand. I believed without a doubt that Nina would regain a normal childhood, but when? I made strategies, set deadlines. Hopes held fast even as horizons shrank. I was captive to three things: the idiosyncratic course of Nina's days, the constant interruptions of my night's sleep, and the loss of an intimate other who could empathize.

Kai was the one with all the freedom, a devoted father ill-equipped for the daily drudgery of it all. In my heart the seed of bitterness grew as I watched him embark for the world of adults and then return home as someone prized in their eyes. That he could not seem to grasp the scope of my day-to-day disappointments drove a wedge that neither of us could budge.

The more Nina grew, the more apparent her difference. I was exiled from the cozy parents' club where women enjoyed watching each other's kids doing the same things. Nina was behind, Nina was recalcitrant, Nina was scared, Nina was disinterested in the shared wonder of the world unfolding. She was missing it, and that meant I missed something, too. Often, after D-Day, pity for myself competed with the heady rush to mobilize on her behalf.

At least we were lucky to have had this child in a time of burgeoning research, feisty demanding parents, and sharp-eyed advocates. The Betty Bolens of the world had the videos and the data to prove that recovery happened. Recovery would be Nina's; I just had to keep shoulder to the wheel.

On the parent list-serves, in the support groups, there was absolutely no truck with depression, self-pity, or despair. We were going to win. Breakthroughs were waiting around the next corner. This epidemic was temporary, so buck up and read the latest book on autism, research your heart out on the Internet, go to a meeting of like-minded parents. I did these things but still felt like a prisoner—of the house, of autism, of my own lack of moorings—and tried to hide it with all my might.

During this time, when women from a state prison wrote looking for a priestess to guide their study of the Goddess, I kept mum about my anger at Her. I wanted to be needed *differently* than Nina needed me, I needed to get out of the house. I could relate to those women's situation in a way I dared not say, because their horrors Inside were the stuff of nightmares. But we shared the commonality of being bound to a physical place, a rigid schedule, and the same faces. Fenced in. Feeling punished.

For a few months I tried to help them, but they couldn't understand my situation and I could hardly press them. I knew they'd take offense if I dared mention that my own life felt like prison. Their needs were too great. Before Nina, during days with my therapy clients, I had been available for the intensity of an I-Thou relationship that was not diluted by the everyday banal. But while parenting Nina I often couldn't muster the energy the women needed in order to face their crises inside the state correctional system. I tried to be their priestess but flopped, even though I gave my role all I had from dwindling re-serves. Trouble was, I'm no actress. They deserved better.

Chapter 13
MOTHER AS STUDENT BODY

It didn't feel like a temple of the soul, let alone a microcosm of the Goddess incarnate. This body I lived in was sick, and it went beyond headaches. I hurt all over.

Was I sick because I was depressed? Was I depressed because I was stressed to the point of ill health? Circles within circles of rationale—I followed them endlessly, destination nowhere.

The situation—marching feminist and former Rebel Girl, tied to her house and domestic duty—lost its amusing irony. I never admitted publicly to feeling sick or depressed, just *tired*. But something was drastically wrong inside my mind.

My good guides had thrown up their hands and left me high and dry. I couldn't make it through a relaxation sequence without either falling asleep or careening off into worry. If I couldn't trance-heal myself, then that ace-in-the-hole for evading the Wohler Madness was gone. Suddenly I was an anxious June Cleaver, minus A-line dress and pearls. No, I was Agnes Wohler Elton, driven mad by grief over all that was lost, all that Nina and I were missing.

What does Chronic Fatigue Syndrome feel like, I wondered? How do you claim it, where was the reliable test? I'd known a woman with the Epstein-Barr virus who could barely venture from her bed. I feared that fate because I knew I *had* to keep moving for my daughter. But it was Herculean, the daily effort. Whenever a migraine hit, I slogged onward with the life-spark drained through some karmic straw.

Would I, like Agnes, embrace this dirty deal as my just desserts? I couldn't give Kai the biological child he craved; surely this was my punishment. The Boones, who gave us Nina, were *my* friends. It was all my fault.

Yet this mysterious child evoked the fiercest love from both of us. Behind Kai's frenetic pace in the work world lay an anguish for Nina too painful for him to hold. We never stopped asking each other, "What is it about her? What is it?" Didn't we see in her the relentless urge, the surge to connect, to learn, to *get it*, whatever it was that we wanted her to?

Especially now that she was coming around, with yeast beasts on the run and food-opiates shown the door.

A brave parent who recovered her autistic boy through the gluten-free, casein-free (GFCF) diet (Karyn Seroussi, author of *Unraveling the Mystery of Autism and PDD: A Mother's Tale of Research and Recovery*) polled her support group and found that fifty percent of the mothers of autistic children had fibromyalgia (FMS), a disease characterized by chronic joint pain and fatigue. A sufferer of FMS herself, she consulted a geneticist who uncovered a number of "red flags"—psychological and neurological disorders running through her family history. But my child was adopted and, since the disappearance of the Boones, we had no access to further medical histories. This was yet another way they'd left Nina high and dry—but what did it mean for me?

It meant that I would be foolish to pass up this opportunity for a double healing, foolish to blame either Boone genetics or the Wohler destiny. There was no way Nina stood to catch anything from the Wohler line, yet here she was with a diagnosis once confused with childhood schizophrenia. Our parallel tracks—so close yet with no shared blood, both of us beset by ailments that halted life as we should have lived it—were far too coincidental.

Nina handed me the perfect opportunity to investigate my family tree for answers.

The first experiment would be performed on me.

❊ ❊ ❊

Kai and I giggled like teenagers. The waiter was coming, but we didn't care what he thought. We were out-of-towners. A night away from the kids!

My parents had gifted us with a stay at a bed and breakfast. Maybe the novelty of being alone together in a fancy restaurant made us laugh at nothing. I reached for the fresh-baked dinner rolls that our server positioned with pride. Two bites, and I headed into the eye-stab of impending migraine.

When most people get a moment of truth after a night on the town, it probably concerns the ill effects of alcohol, not a fluffy crescent roll. But that night I was like an addict who'd had it: I finally swore off wheat.

Nina, of course, had been gluten-free for over a year. We found that wheat flour had some substitutes like brown rice flour, workable in pasta, cereals, and other staples. These substitutes cost more, so they were reserved for Nina's stash of special foods. Or that's how I rationalized my continuing gluten gluttony.

My love affair with bread was as intense as the cheese fixation. Like many a hippie gal, I'd taught myself to knead and tend wholegrain dough, munching down half a loaf soon after it came steaming from the oven. Rejection of wheat was heresy for a Kansan, where the harvest is a major cultural event.

On the Finley farm I rode horses knee-high into its waving glory. When I turned to mythology for spirit-balm, I learned that in ancient times the Son of the Goddess was incarnate as the grain itself. In the agri-bizzed heartland of North America, that meant hard red winter wheat. I'd stop by fields to clip a handful for the seasonal altar. Reverence, habit, and economics were all tied together when it came to this grain that was native to neither American nor European soil. Wheat in the wild is nearly inedible, and cultivation never solved the problems we encountered when ingesting the domesticated version.

It turns out that the grain isn't easy on human digestion: the gluten molecules resist breaking down. What's left are "peptide chains" too long—and too toxic—for the lining of the intestine. These chains cause serious inflammation, a smashing down of important cells that need to be rough-and-ready against foreigners on their way to the bloodstream. This in turn prompts an immune response. Basically, the body attacks itself.

That night when I swore off wheat, all I knew was that I ate it and then I hurt. Although it felt like I was losing a great friend, I tried to put on a brave face. I made it through our all-too-brief vacation somehow. I didn't want Kai to start in on me for ruining things, the way he did whenever he saw the telltale squint in my right eye that meant a migraine was moving in. Years of watching me succumb on a regular basis had left him feeling helpless. When in pain, all I wanted was to be held, to inhale the scent of my lover, warmed by his warmth. Too often that wasn't possible in a life with a kid, life with autism. It was a trick even to find time to relax together, let alone embrace. I would be hard pressed to say that we were close, a relative term in marriage.

Our days were strained by efforts such as prying services out of the recalcitrant school district or shouldering a second mortgage and numerous lines of credit. Kai worked harder at his career to cover what the health insurance shirked and did his best to parent around the edges.

We labored to keep hope alive and sustained ourselves on Nina's progress, which was considerable since starting the GFCF diet and taming her yeast beasts. Our couch potato was now a mover. She had words, she had the motivation to make us understand her, though primarily we still existed as agents to fill her needs.

Goodbye, amber waves

So now it was my turn. I had everything to learn from my daughter. While Nina experienced the ban on dairy first, I went backwards: first the wheat and no cheat. Maybe I'd squeak through with barley, oats, and rye—keep some familiar gods intact, hold onto my milk and cream cheese for a while (I'd heard that aged cheeses worsen PMS, so I'd dropped them long ago). I couldn't go cold turkey on cow-tit, not yet.

However, I was forced to cut those ties in short order. These sensitivities are a highly individualized matter, and some people may not be able to get by with a nip here and there. It takes only a few molecules to create one opioid from casein or gluten, so there's a lot of bang in a bite. Given the morphine-like effect, the addictive urge is activated—and the next bite is harder to resist. I'm not strong enough, and the risk isn't worth it.

Perhaps the opiate effect of food (spike, then crash) explains why it takes so long to wise up, to admit that what you eat is involved in the process of madness. It's so much more poetic to ponder the madness-genius link as a holy mystery. No one wants to believe that their personal story of emotional havoc can be traced to the mundane door of something they ate. "Bad doughnut," Kai quipped when I missed his company party due to a migraine. His listeners cackled, figuring me a slacker. Food poisoning was one thing, food allergy a somewhat frivolous excuse.

If they'd been in my shoes, they'd have known what I knew: withdrawal was hell.

Any bit of gluten set in motion that wrecking ball to the skull. Not just wheat, but good old barley soup was nixed; no more brown, caraway-flecked rye bread, either. Oats were a maybe, but I didn't press. I was getting paranoid about any gluten-bearer.

When Kai prepared his famous cinnamon rolls right under my nose, it was downright traumatic. I never could have stuck to this diet without a powerful aversive: the mean monster migraine, where the voices I heard were not so different from those my brother Sam attributed to strangers. The sniper talk was clearly on the inside, but still I questioned the bare facts: you're only lying still in a dark room because you have a *headache*?

What I really *had* constituted so much more than that. Migraine was an usher for the agents of inner sabotage to seize control with no Os, no thorough understanding of my child's illness, for balance.

I would eat nothing but brown rice if it meant getting rid of the self-hater that suffocates, that plays back any number of life-mistakes in review: wince, cringe, try to block it out, then onto the next. I never believed (nor did those spiteful internal voices tell me) that I was schizophrenic. Only I was something worse: defective. Marked by the Wohler legacy—maybe not madness, but a fear that led to missing out on what others seemed to manage with aplomb. An underachiever via a gene design that had caused faulty choices over decades. Not normal, yet not strange enough to get to Yr.

If I could no longer connect to the Goddess through trance and ceremony, at least She was alive and well in my kitchen. I discovered a world of new grains—quinoa, amaranth, millet, teff—and learned strange new tricks needed to cook GFCF such as xanthum gum (fluffs up baked goods) and arrowroot thickener. When I converted one of my favorite rye flatbreads into a tasty alternative, Nina begged for crackers made with garbanzo-bean flour. Who knew? Flour out of beans!

Betty Bolen was gathering recipes for a GFCF cookbook at the time, and I presented her with my Soft and Sweet Chocolate Chip Cookies, made with an alternative herbal sweetener, stevia, a sugar that doesn't feed candida yeast. In fact there were a number of moms sharing on the Internet, and with their own self-published cookbooks for sale at conferences, they seemed bent on approximating most classics of the All-American diet done gluten and casein (dairy) free. Confession: I'm not the most inventive cook, and their recipes were essential. Our family found we could still eat the likes of pizza, fish sticks, mashed potatoes, even ice cream. When I visited a health-food store and found a new food that Nina could enjoy, a food I'd loved as a kid, I could be found in the aisle literally wiping away tears. The afternoon I came across GFCF Oreos I was awash in gratitude; drinking my first glass of hemp milk, Nina's favorite, I experienced a mouth-feel almost as creamy as the real thing.

Yet some comfort foods simply remained impossible. There was no macaroni and cheese homemade or store bought that wasn't dull or disgusting. Try as I might, I couldn't find a biscuit recipe that came close. I recall having friends over for pie, and the crust was so hard we joked about eating the filling and flying our Frisbees. But there was no turning back.

I was fighting for someone else now. Nina was here, and I wouldn't give up on her the way my parents gave up on me.

Nor would I die trying to save her. If I was too sick, how could I help Nina?

But I was coming around to a truth about the Wohler malady. Without Nina, I would never have seen it. Food just might be making me crazy, fatigued, anti-social. I would follow my daughter's lead on health, down to the molecular level, casting every opiate in the trash bin.

After going completely GFCF, I was migraine-free for six weeks. I hurt less all over and took much more of the day's stress in stride. I lost considerable weight (though I was slim by nature, after being a little bit pregnant four times and a whole lot depressed, that had changed).

New to "pounding it on" in midlife, my shame was deep. Banishing wheat and dairy products relieved me of that burden—about thirty pounds worth.

Yet by far the greatest prize was mental, not physical. There was something to this after all—and not just for a person with autism. The biggest surprise, coming in only a week's time, was the tapering off of the constant, horrid self-talk—the kind where you lose time, real time, in rewinding all you should have said, or blurted out when you shouldn't have. Self-judgments that make you want to hide your face from the neighbors or lash out at a spouse who must be defective for loving you.

Whole categories of negative thought patterns vanished into thin air. I quit worrying about the stupid thing I'd just said to the clerk, the bus driver, or the husband. I wondered if in fact I was speaking more to the point—more directly but without the edginess. At the same time the future started filling in, with brave possibilities assuaging the bleak void.

Waiting for the other shoe to drop, I wondered if the self-hater might have the real goods on my truly ugly core, where I deserved what I got. But if that was the case, then who was this GFCF person living free of inner bad-mouthing? How could I say she was a fake, when she was such a clear-cut improvement? How real then could that anxious one be who, before the diet, always reached for Excedrin to mute the chorus of naysayers inside?

The migraines did return, but came much less frequently. I was hopeful. Surely there was a stone unturned somewhere and I would find it. Maybe it wasn't only the kid who could recover.

Nina was now talking, using one word request-commands like *juice, pasta* (rice bran, of course), *car.* Her repertoire expanded weekly as she took on the behaviorists' tasks of matching colors with shapes and learning their names. Books, her great love, were examined appropriately, page-by-page. And oh, could she carry a tune! Although the words were inarticulate, Nina's memory for melodies ranging from Lynyrd Skynyrd to Bach was forever. Whenever Nina sang, Kai and I stopped what we were doing, the moment suspended by her certain gift and that unspoken word: *savant.*

The fungus among us

What was Nina's next lesson for me? The beasts that were known as yeast.

Here was another powerful weapon that we deployed ruthlessly against autism as we slowly let go of milky love and Kansas grain. Giving yeast the heave-ho was accomplished with a prescription drug called Nystatin. It was a relatively benign concoction and the results showed up within a week.

Nina and I were rocking on that same front porch where she once laughed at nothing in the corners. We sat in her favorite chair with Nina in her usual back-to-me position. Suddenly she reclined into my arms, looked directly into my eyes, and smiled. She actually saw me rather than seeing through me, and she was glad. So was I!

"Welcome back, little girl!"

These are the capsules of time we hold close. When she emerges. When she enjoys.

When she connects. Within days Nina was running up and down the driveway again, moving about the world.

Death to the yeast!

When it was my turn, my biggest reticence concerned the yeast die-off period. Hadn't my daughter had a rough ride during it? Could I afford several days of getting worse—how much worse? I read all I could find on the beasts of gut-yeast, and knew they had me under their spell.

Beyond playing a part in autism, I discovered that candida overgrowth plays a role in a wide range of health problems beyond fatigue and headaches. It can worsen the likes of asthma, psoriasis, multiple sclerosis, Crohn's disease, lupus, heart disease, stroke, cancer, AIDS, and infertility. *Infertility!* I shuddered at what I wished I'd known earlier.

The herbal preparation Biocidin had become Nina's mainstay after we realized that Nystatin would not attack all the harmful gut bugs living in her intestinal tract. I ordered my own bottle. But I was too reckless. I kept going full speed, didn't ingest enough immune support, and got a whooping bad cold, the first in years. I fortified myself with the thought that at least I hadn't diagnosed wrong; something was going on, even if initially it was a shaky ride.

At the end of the tunnel, there was more than light. Two weeks of traveling through the badlands, if it meant getting safely home, was worth it. Not a migraine surfaced during this time, and I was certain I had them on the run by now. Going GFCF chased some surly tenants out of the mind, followed by a whole new crowd I was pleased to see moving in.

Clarity. Energy. Optimism.

Thought patterns turned more benign without me prodding them or expending conscious energy "working on myself." I would suddenly notice the change, and smile. Scaffolds of negative thinking about self and others collapsed in a heap. There was more room in my mind, it seemed. The clutter was gone, the focus sharpening.

It wasn't that I'd finally found true immunity or fail-proof escape from the Wohler Madness. Rather, the family disease had been exposed, renamed, and dismantled, transformed from stigma-sprouting blame game into a clear science of minding the gut. I saw our supposed genetic curse for what it always was, at least in this flesh: the missed body-mind connection. *Not* the other way around, with a sick mind twisting biology into illness and pain.

This challenged some long-held assumptions about the need for lifelong psychotherapy in a person like me. How would I ever make my way back to the consulting room, the incredibly charged vessel of therapy?

Unfortunately, these revelations also threw some cold water on my convictions about magic and trance.

Goodbye guides

I was ready for my guides' return, certain of reunion now that my head was finally clear. But beloved Os and the others failed to show.

Not that they'd been much help in the face of autism. I considered that my fault, since I could never relax. But in the wake of my gut-based epiphany, the very urge toward trance, toward meeting the guides, had changed. I wanted to "see" them…yet at the same time it seemed pedestrian. Without these guides, who would I be?

Minus cow and grain, minus the beasts of a yeasty gut, I felt tons better. I was able to return to trance, to focus, let go, and deepen down. But it was an empty awareness. Where was everybody? Who was present? Just me. It was unsettling, but I wasn't going back. There was a quality to waking reality that hadn't been there before. Meaning that I was more awake. It was more than bearable, now, to be alive.

The shift in body chemistry that came after kicking the bad-mood foods affected more than my mind. I still felt estranged from the Goddess, and the hole without a spiritual practice hurt. But changing the foods that sustained me also began to change my attitude toward consciousness. Enter the Buddhist concept of "mindfulness."

Why would I want an extra dose of the here and now? If anybody needed escape, surely it was me. Yet the symbolism of magic felt like so much distraction on the way to the good stuff, the ever-present awareness of the everyday. With Nina on the mend and my mind opening to what it could have been from the start, I continued to marvel. Chronic body aches disappeared and the need for the cherished nap became a thing of the past. It allowed me to contemplate the next step, which forays into meditation helped to make clear. My task was to break free from resentment over infertility, autism, isolation. The key was compassion for self and others, or I would surely drown.

Parenting a child with a severe disability made the need to de-stress paramount. Mindfulness meditation promised results. "Stop striving," advised the tapes and books I collected on the topic. "Only *observe* the mind. Note the breath. Mind wanders? Begin again." What a relief: there was no way to fail, no intrinsic talent required. If you get off track, you simply *begin again*.

The effects surprised me. A letting go *and* a taking in that was much like the visitation of the osprey during the New Age hypnosis seminar. A widening of view. Since time for regular meditation was spotty, my practice was to test the lessons of mindfulness while engaged in everyday living. I went about the business of parenting, studying autism, advocating for Nina with the following concerns: How present can I be? How is loving-kindness called for here? How fully can one heart explore the freedom to *begin again*? And still I kept asking myself why was I finally able to meditate, and why were trance-journeys now a crushing bore?

During this period I read a novel called *Lying Awake* by Mark Salzer. The protagonist is a cloistered nun flung between health issues and visionary experience. Searing headaches bring her ecstatic visions of God, and in between attacks she writes about and publishes her encounters. She learns that surgery promises relief, which implies that her illness is responsible for—and the operation thus likely to sever—the mystical connection. Which is real? Which to choose?

In my case, after decades of painful migraines, the choice was clear. My headaches brought only self-torturing criticisms and moved me farther from any sense of what might be termed Divine. It may be true that the extraordinary trance experiences I had were made possible through a brain constantly swirling with food opiates. Though it took a long time to connect the dots between migraine, food allergies, and candidiasis, I made a pact to trust my gut and embrace food without highs.

Pill poppers

Kai entered the kitchen to fetch his coffee on the way to court and said, "Well, if it isn't the Supplement Queen." I was in the process of raiding Nina's stash for myself, juggling several capsules in one hand while fiddling with another bottle. "This ups the bill," he grumbled down the hall.

But it wasn't long before he was downing his own handful morning and night.

If only there were one pill to treat autism! Any number of sedatives were available from a doctor's office, but since we found it difficult to call Nina crazy we never considered anti-depressants or neuroleptics. Anything that Samuel might now or ever have been on felt as creepy as insulin coma or electroshock.

Enter the vitamin and supplement routines...way too many of them to choose from. Family doctors were no help, but with luck we, like other parents in our shoes, found Defeat Autism Now (DAN).

There were two doctors in the Kansas City area to steer one's course, both of them DAN doctors. DAN is a determined and organized lot of practitioners and researchers of every stripe who bucked the credo of No Cure by believing otherwise. They hold lively conferences, share information and, best of all, listen to parents.

So along with The Diet came the supplements suggested by the DAN doctors. I'd taken vitamin C and B-complex for years, but the true extent of nutrient therapy was a new world. Why did Nina need all of these supplements? Partly because The Diet, plus her famous food-pickiness, meant that key nutrients were missing from her meals. Not so different, really, from those of us running on Hamburger Helper and Diet Coke—but autism, according to the DAN findings, entailed a ravaged gut, immune dysfunction, and endocrine issues, plus synthetic chemical and heavy metal overload with the inability to detoxify the same. What system in the body *wasn't* under attack?

The problem? No mass blueprint existed to guide necessary treatment. Each autistic child was uniquely damaged. Could that also be true for persons with so-called mental illness? Could it be the same for me, battling anxious depression and mystery fatigue?

I listened to the DAN movers and shakers with an ear out for what might help Nina or me. I talked to other parents, but mostly I just tried stuff. Such are the experiments of modern-day alchemists, mixing relative unknowns in the flasks of our children's bodies and our own, going for the gold of health and a recovery that would return the spirit to one's life.

In the beginning, the entity we called "Big Pharma" could have cared less—vitamins were poor relations, and hardly a threat. Pharmaceutical companies weren't yet under fire for raking in huge profits while many other industries faltered, for using their money on new designer drugs and getting their favored candidates into Congress. Still and all, when it came to medicine, Pharma had the mighty fusion reactors (never mind the side effects) while vitamins and supplements were the windmills and solar panels. For parents who felt their children were forgotten, our allies were each other, the Internet, and the nearest natural food store.

Kai saw in time that the supplements were working for Nina in all the key areas: speech, sociability, calm, and ability to learn. Her development was slow but steady and never stalled.

I felt as though we were on a quest for the Holy Grail: a recovered daughter. Kai and I talked about it a great deal, about the day Nina would be well. We believed. Our faith was reckless and born of searing pain inside that tender, first-time-parent's heart. Nina would be well, and we would look back on this from the land where the Grail winner lives in perfect love and perfect trust. There were nights when I dreamed she was talking to me. I hated to wake up.

Every time one of her supplements worked favorably on my body-mind, too, it was one more victorious step. Meanwhile, there were many knights we encountered along the quest; across the divide of parent and professional, we knew one another as fellows caught up in the search. They were allergists, osteopaths, naturopaths, speech therapists, occupational therapists, physical therapists, and more therapists, each with their cherished angle. Most of them urged more of what they had to give as the key to the cure. What else did we expect them to say? Every treatment cost a lot of money. So Kai worked even harder. He took more supplements. We pressed on, with visions of the finish line as our reason to get up in the morning.

Chapter 14
HEROES UNSUNG

Kai was in town buying groceries. I hung out with Nina, watching a *Baby Einstein* video. Suddenly her eyes shut and stayed shut. Then a river of drool, a cascade beyond typical baby spit that seemed to flow forever. Nina was immobile, arms at her sides, a likeness of herself on hold. It lasted twenty seconds at most.

I freaked and called the paramedics, then had Kai paged at the store to speed home. Two young guys in an ambulance arrived, but by then Nina was back in fine form. She seemed happier. They took her vital signs as I recounted the details.

"She had a seizure," said the lanky one, handing Nina a small stuffed witch with a sweet, Strawberry Shortcake look. "Probably what they call 'grand mal,'" he added.

"*Grand?* But there was no jerking all over the place, no swallowing the tongue…"

"The petit mal is just a split-second blackout," he said, packing up. "You gonna be all right?"

"My husband's on his way. Why did this happen? What do we do?"

"Call a pediatric neurologist. You'll have to go to Kansas City."

Back to the teaching hospital for us. Oh, joy.

As Nina stood close to the TV screen, tapping on the cavorting characters, I kept thinking, *First autistic, now epileptic. This can't be happening.*

Embattled brains

Another frustrating afternoon of waiting for Godot—that is, the specialist of high repute. A three-hour wait, in fact. Parents were going ballistic in the packed lobby, and the reception room staff could do little besides barricade themselves behind tight lips. Every once in a while someone cracked, and you heard the voice of hysteria demanding to know when, for crying out loud, would the doctor be ready for them? Nina, testy as the next neurologically damaged kid-in-tow, clung to me to block out the noise and swelter.

When it was our turn, it felt like winning the lottery. But we merely walked down the hall and waited another hour in a little examining room. *Doctors' Cubicles R Us*, I thought. Finally the aging, anorexic-looking neurologist entered, reeking of money and liquor. She looked so frail and apologetic that we made no fuss about the pressurized compartments we'd been subjected to. She listened to everything we knew about Nina's seizures, which were coming randomly now every few days, sometimes several days in a row.

The neurologist asked Nina to build a tower of blocks. *Uh oh, here it comes.* I knew Kai was on the same thought-wave, breath held for an early verdict. When Nina nimbly placed one block on top of the other and the tower held, we gasped. The nice lady doctor then ordered an EEG and bowed out.

Results: inconclusive. Definite epileptiform patterns in her brain, but too early to pin down the E-word. Take this, said the neurologist, it's called Depokene. Thus the industry known as Pharma stepped into our lives.

The medicine made Nina a zombie. Her seizures continued unabated.

Nothing, it seemed, applied anymore.

On my headboard I placed a picture of Kali Durga, a can-do divinity of India, her many arms brandishing the implements of her goddess-nature. Her face is serene amidst all that needs doing. With her sword, trident, and lotus, she is called upon by the other gods to dispatch a plague of demons. But did She speak to me, did I feel She cared? With my new interest in mindfulness, still feeling sold out by the Goddess, Asian or Hindu deities were about as close as I'd get to the Divine. Kali Durga's face was no more than a mnemonic device, a reminder to persevere inside the whirlwind. Apparently I no longer deserved a juicy, guiding Moon Goddess in my life.

This crisis of faith was embarrassing because I knew better. Turning bitter towards the Unseen over bad luck was too much like the biblical Book of Job, where God and the devil conspire to hound a man with misfortune to see at what point he forsakes his faith. My Goddess didn't demand allegiance. She was no sugar-mama, dispensing whatever I wanted just because I called Her name.

On better days, I accepted the notion that being tested to the extreme was a fact of family life. Such trials were a consequence of asking for more soul development. I put myself in a position to grow up and the Universe, or *Whoever*, was taking me up on it.

Nina was as confused and scared as I was, and in far greater pain. She couldn't journal, meditate, turn to a partner, or even tell anyone what was wrong. When she clung to me, I was a life raft with a big responsibility. She was not stuck within herself by choice; on the outside she looked intact, but she lacked the tools for growth and relationship. She wanted relief, she wanted peace, and she deserved the basics: communication, understanding, plus a calm gut and brain.

Fears about Nina's seizures became all consuming. When her eyelids slammed shut and sounds choked on the misfires in her nervous system, I became the Ultimate Inadequate. I could do nothing to change the course of the event nor could I prevent the next one—I could not even imagine it, let alone accompany her. The worst dread of all was that I knew the seizures were debilitating, taking a toll on her body's systems, robbing her vital force little by little.

Then we heard about blue-green algae from the Klamath Lake in Oregon and its beneficial effects on children with ADHD. The first day we gave some to Nina, she acted wound-up tighter than an eight-day clock. That night she scurried about the house, darting from room to room in a display of hyper that wasn't her style, pushing her big green exercise ball—then had a massive seizure, and went right to bed.

It was her last seizure for an entire year. That was also the year she slept soundly through the night.

Kai and I praised the plant microorganisms from an ecosystem far from our prairie knowledge, blue-green like the planet on which we play out our lives. Ah, eight straight hours in which to dream! No more worrying whether Nina might fall off the swing set if she seizured, whether sitters were prepared to handle it, whether we could live with the looming diagnosis of epilepsy on the way to the Grail.

Precursors

My endless search for helpful information uncovered yet another researcher with a different take on the problem, one that appeared to go to a genetically based root. It struck a chord with me.

While R.D. Laing geared up to become the prophet of a psychedelic psychiatry, a Canadian psychiatrist was musing on the connection between hallucinogens and madness. His name was Dr. Abram Hoffer and, in 1951, he and colleagues began looking at all known hallucinogens with this premise: in the bodies of some persons there is a madness-inducing toxin on the rampage that results in schizophrenia.

The doctors confirmed that when adrenalin oxidizes, it turns pink (also known as adrenochrome); they also confirmed that it is made in the body, it is hallucinogenic, and that shutting down its formation should be a top priority in the treatment of schizophrenics. But how?

The group turned to user-friendly a B-3 vitamin, niacin. In double-blind studies, a majority of patients (early diagnosed, not chronic, and followed up for two years) recovered. The experiment improved Pharma's 35 percent recovery rate to 75 percent.

But the groundbreaking news came too late—the drug companies were already on the move. Tranquilizers were in, quick and easy. Psychiatrists tested the effectiveness of the new drugs by using a noise meter on psychotic wards. Ah, suddenly patients were quiet! Success! The drugs were proclaimed a godsend. (By the way, they were patented, which Vitamin B-3 could never be.)

Pressured by employers growing embarrassed over his work with vitamins, in 1967 Hoffer resigned his post as chief government researcher and professor of medicine. He longed to be of real service and chose private practice. Although he never intended to see children, a few were referred to him. The good doctor was astounded when large doses of Vitamin B-3, along with mega doses of Vitamin C, markedly improved the childhood behavior disorders that increasingly brought patients to him for evaluation. Meticulous follow-up confirmed the results.

Soon Dr. Hoffer made the acquaintance of Linus Pauling, and Orthomolecular Psychiatry was born.

Meanwhile, in Princeton, New Jersey, yet another physician became involved in psychiatric research. As a young medical student, he began to suspect the role of nutritional imbalance in mental illness. For thirteen years, until the state withdrew funds for the research, he developed biochemical tests to identify diverse types of schizophrenia. His name was Carl Pfeiffer.

Dr. Pfeiffer's interests quickly broadened to hypoglycemia (low blood sugar), arthritis, food allergies, digestive disorders, and heavy metal poisoning. Parents on the Internet were buzzing about his namesake institution, the Pfeiffer Treatment Center.

Sometimes I'd get a whole-body radar wave that told me when a particular treatment could make a humongous difference for Nina. Deep in my bones, I knew we should take her to the Pfeiffer Treatment Center near Chicago.

If Kai was devastated because Nina would never achieve academically, would always be a financial burden, and couldn't walk in his professional footsteps, he never expressed it in words. His depth of feeling for her was unchanged, but his confidence as a provider was challenged. We didn't have the funds to whisk her to every newly promising treatment center with the newest angle on autism. Plus it was in his legally trained nature to beware of flimflammers at every turn.

But by the Goddess, and despite his misgivings, we flew to Chicago for a full work-up by the intellectual descendants of one of the great, unheralded scientists of our time.

Silence in Boone-ville and a ray of hope

Kai and I fretted that Nina would fall apart in airports and airplanes. The noise! The smells! The sensations of takeoff and landing! But other than signaling us to carry her small frame through the crowds, she did remarkably well. She often stumped us like that. There's no standard pattern to the sensory sensitivity of a person with autism. They may not bat an eye at a roaring blender, but scream at the slightest jangle of car keys. Despite the many sounds that could set her off, Nina's urge to go places was stronger.

She seemed to find the jet hop to Chicago interesting, and we were pleased to have her between us, sipping juice at her tray table. Kai read a newspaper while I talked to Nina about the clouds and went over the forms for the Pfeiffer docs. As usual, there was not much to tell about the birth family tree. By then, I was used to writing "N/A—child is adopted." Aidan was silent when I telephoned him for more information. Pages came back blank through our fax machine. What *was* their problem, anyway?

Toxins on parade

The Pfeiffer Treatment Center was in a low, spreading building in what appeared to be a banal suburb—part industrial, part office park—with many chain restaurants. Its waiting room offered a comfortable family clinic with the usual clutter of toys, magazines, and sturdy furniture. At the reception counter, a copy of *Natural Healing for Schizophrenia* by Eva Edelson was prominently displayed. My heart leaped for Samuel. Could this place help him, too?

Although Nina had already drooled through three seizures that week, the plane ride passed without incident. Her ease in making the trip allowed me to focus on this new healing environment.

Called in by a smiling nurse, we steered Nina through the halls to intake interviews, blood draws, vital signs and other tests—the usual, or perhaps a bit more. Yet what hallways these were! More than mere passageways for conducting clinic business, each wall sported large-print, floor-to-ceiling research abstracts and data showing results of a very provocative nature. The Pfeiffer clinic clearly had an urgent message to share.

While Nina was ministered to, I stood before the text, stunned.

The Pfeiffer specialists had been studying more than just children. They'd examined blood samples from serial killer Charles Manson, a disgruntled postal worker who gunned down fellow employees, and other famed murderers. The results, published first in peer-reviewed journals, were writ large in these halls for all to see: serial killers and other violent criminals were loaded with toxic metals and nutrient imbalances far beyond the general population.

Spelled out in language Friedrich Wohler would have prized, the walls of the Pfeiffer Treatment Center offered an explanation for the escalating violence of humankind.

My skin prickled at the scope of the implications. Killers were monsters, weren't they? Not like us, or our children, although perhaps they were horribly abused as kids or twisted by poverty? Looking at the research, however, I was pushed to do more than add another do-gooder excuse to the list of reasons why people could turn out so horribly wrong.

This finding went beyond autism, even beyond mental health. Why wasn't the nutrient angle being explored as a way to address the animosity that preoccupied our world, especially our adolescents? No town, it seemed, was immune: one Easter Sunday, in the middle of quiet Kansas, two junior high students set the elementary school on fire. Kai himself had served as counsel for a trio of boys who had played with guns to disastrous results. What was the juvenile justice system to do?

Had the intellectual descendants of Carl Pfeiffer discovered the cause of all the chaos, crime, and conflict in the United States? Were people toxic as hell?

Finally it was our turn with the beautiful Dr. Uppal. She was focused yet tranquil, reminding me of the Indian deity Kali Durga with her many tasks, her many tools in hand. There was, of course, nothing definitive to be said about Nina without test results, but she made sure we'd heard about the copper-zinc imbalance theory. Dr. Uppal couldn't pinpoint anything yet but reiterated the odds that Nina was similarly afflicted.

We returned to the airport at night. Now that I'd heard Pfeiffer's exposé, metal gleamed everywhere like a new menace, no longer the workhorse taken for granted. Cars streaking down the asphalt, the enormous billboards towering over the highway, and even the tube soon to rise into the air were all metal. Tiny wires in the medical machinery we'd just left behind could have been copper, a menace when overloaded into brains and bodies. Metal buttresses the world, a solid holder and helper, a conductor, shelter, and strength. Reliable and strong, it gets things done. What was the alternative—a life of lumber and cloth?

Epilepsy outwitted

"This is easy. This is nice." Kai was opening two giant capsules from a big prescription bottle and dumping the contents into juice. They were Nina's, from the Pfeiffer compounding pharmacy. Everything already mixed together, no time-consuming unscrewing bottles from this or that company.

"I'll tell you what's nicer," I began. He looked at me, eyebrows on the rise. I knew what he was thinking: *Don't say it—it might go away.* "Knock on wood—she's been seizure-free ever since that stuff came. It's been a month."

"I wouldn't rejoice yet," he said.

"Then when?"

"Well, she went a year on the algae before the seizures started again."

"Do I have to wait a year to claim a victory? You just don't get how parched I am for good news. I need to jump up and down on more than an annual basis."

"Then knock yourself out. Maybe it'll work. Those folks at Pfeiffer didn't seem like crackpots, and I have to admit the girl is talking more."

"Not just talking more. Connecting more. She's lucid. She's present. It's like she's joined our family."

We locked eyes. Kai reached up and gathered my long hair with one hand, then curved it over my shoulder with the other.

It was a lost sign of tenderness from the olden days.

PART FOUR
LUNACY'S LAST STAND

Chapter 15
HEAVY METAL MADNESS

Our first seminar about autism seemed so long ago. Back then, parent-researcher Betty Bolen had said something about immunizations causing the disorder. It seemed far-fetched. What did she want, people dying like flies from horrible epidemics? More plausible villains were the antibiotics prescribed like candy for countless infections—and disturbing the flora in Nina's bowels. But one's programming is geared toward trusting medical authorities, not toward asking questions.

Yet a stronger wind was blowing about theories of autism recovery, and we were ready to be propelled. The GFCF diet, the supplements: they managed symptoms, but never got to the root cause. If the beneficent bovine and the golden grain turned suspect, that was one thing—the solution was to avoid them.

But what if malevolency lurked in one of the more altruistic movements of modern times, like the push to vaccinate against childhood diseases? What better-intentioned public health initiative existed in the world? This was far worse than going up against Wonder Bread and a glass of milk.

I vaguely remembered hippie parents who didn't vaccinate. They never explained it, or maybe I wasn't motivated to listen back then. Days after we brought Nina home, Sandra Boone urged us to get her immunized. Were we unsure whether the birth parents had her up-to-date? No matter, give them again, it can't hurt! I felt contentedly normal holding my baby on my lap while a professional white-coat punctured her skin.

Did I notice any adverse reaction? Was I even looking? No reason to doubt this cornerstone of preventive health. Kai and I chalked up Nina's off moments—and her foul explosive poops, her aloofness, her nonstop ear infections, her delays at accomplishing this, that, or the other milestone—to the birth family genes. We adamantly did not want to hear about trouble with immunizations.

Eventually, I came across the work of Dr. Andrew Wakefield, a British gastroenterologist whose caseload and research pointed a finger at the Measles, Mumps, and Rubella (MMR) vaccine. After receiving this particular "jab" at 12-18 months of age, many entirely normal toddlers "go away" almost overnight. The change is sudden and dramatic, usually accompanied by reactions to the shot such as fever, screaming, sleeplessness. And *seizures.*

Indeed, we first began to notice Nina's profound lethargy and lack of eye contact during the months following her first MMR shot. She never said "Daddy" again; her tantrums lengthened. Three months after her two-year-old "well baby" visit, replete with more shots such as the DPT, the seizures began.

At a conference in Des Moines, Iowa, I sat through one of Dr. Wakefield's early (yet thoroughly documented) presentations, feeling a morbid new dawn sweep across the room. He spoke of the live measles virus creating autoimmune reactions that were responsible for autistic behavior. But what could be done? The virus might be wreaking havoc in Nina's gut, but it was too late. Apparently, the resulting gastrointestinal pain and immune disruption could never be cured.

More nefarious than food

The mood among autism parents shifted. *Now* what were we going to do, other than stop vaccinating? That didn't seem like the wisest choice, although many decided to pull the plug. Without fanfare, Kai and I followed suit—*just in case.* No more, until they're guaranteed safe. Because what else was in the shots? The discovery was daunting.

Formaldehyde. Aluminum. (Yikes. One of Friedrich Wohler's major achievements was the extraction of aluminum.) Antifreeze, MSG, monkey lung, and kidney cells. Plus the live viruses. Nina received her MMR just four days after her first birthday—completing Year One of an assault on her blood-brain barrier, as yet unformed. And there was yet another substance injected into newborns and infants with no apparent concern: mercury, the second most toxic chemical known to human beings.

Mercury was present in most vaccines in the form of thimerosal, a preservative that soon became a household word on the autism parents' e-mail lists. Thimerosal—it allows for storing several vaccine doses together, which is more efficient and economical for the makers and the jabbers—is 51 percent ethyl mercury.

The problem was that somebody, somewhere in those gargantuan secret societies known best by encryption (CDC, FDA, EPA, VAERS) neglected to do the math. It didn't take a lot of mercury to affect a baby and set her up for learning disabilities, even autism, especially with the blood-brain barrier not yet fully formed. Each time a new vaccine was added to the schedule, the EPA limit of 0.1 microgram per kilogram sounded harmless enough. Yet even the smallest babies, who might weigh only half as much as the largest, received the same amount. Some infants received up to 14 vaccines in one day, making their cumulative dose of mercury *90-240 times* the daily limit, or the equivalent of eight months of daily exposure.

I thought back to my own routine fevers and chills. It was a childhood rite of passage to fall ill with measles, mumps, and chicken pox. Unpleasant, but ah, those lazy days home from school. My mother rose to the occasion—Sam and I were pampered with chicken soup and 7Up, plied with aspirin, and given free rein at the TV. It was a vacation complete with servant, which made the physical discomfort worth it. Heat, red skin, and sore throats were but a speed bump on the fast track to resuming days of play.

Then, vaccination played a role in the community: it was a bona fide event. Whole families lined up with neighbors trailing down the block from the elementary school across the street. It wasn't a Catholic school like mine, and although I'd played on its ball fields and jungle gym countless times, getting inside the lunchroom of the infidels was a scary treat. *En masse* we filed in to receive sugar cubes inoculated with the polio vaccine. Big Brother was keeping us safe.

Forty years later, the vaccine schedule had quadrupled. Still, vaccines as the cause of autism sounded so grim—and I simply couldn't stand the guilt. Childless and clueless, I should have listened to the cautions, but I was skeptical about what sounded like doctor-phobia, if not outright conspiracy theory.

This, plus a lack of confidence in the birth family's genetics, made me view the work of Amy Holmes and Stephanie Cave as the radical fringe I hoped was wrong. These two physicians from Baton Rouge were finding enormous amounts of mercury in their patients. Dr. Holmes had brought her own son out of autism through chelation, the use of prescription compounds to extract toxic metals from deep in the body's tissues. But we'd already had a hair analysis done on Nina (snip a little clip close to the neck and send it to the lab to be tested for metals) and the mercury reading was not so bad.

Mrs. Mercury Mom

I heard more about our own local "mercury mom" one day when I was downtown distributing flyers for an autism support group. A salesperson in one of the shops mentioned that Karen Carnes was suing vaccine manufacturers on behalf of her mercury-poisoned, autistic son. It turned out that I was in Karen's store; Karen, however, wasn't there.

I wasn't exactly sure why I took the flyers. Would I even attend the meeting? I never fit in at these parent support gatherings. I was older, my kid was adopted—and I was too weird for these suburban folk, who appeared normal but for a certain disoriented tint, as if this were the first trauma ever to touch their lives. But this time I reasoned that if I could overlook appearances so could they. I needed a tribe in the worst way and hoped a common anguish would unite us.

Unfortunately, I had a stress-stoked habit of talking too much about topics others preferred to keep personal: *How do you **feel** in the midst of this epidemic? What do you do to take care of yourself?* I embarrassed the other parents and often found myself speaking to dead air, which made it hard to go back. Karen Carnes, I was to find out, avoided most support groups too—but for a different reason. She had bigger fish to fry.

We met for coffee days later. Her voice purred smoothly southern, and Karen took few pains to hide her dislike for Kansas. It was clear that Mr. Mercury Mom was in the doghouse for bringing the family to Osage End. Karen spent her days on the information highway, blocking out the native prairie that lay on the other side of her tall privacy fence.

She was unshakable in her conviction that ethyl mercury in vaccines caused autism. Her lawsuit began years ago, and would take years more to resolve. That didn't bother her. Justice was on the side of her son; in the meanwhile, she channeled her heartbreak into action. She was on a first-name basis with senators, media pundits, and anti-vaccine activists around the U.S. Her fax machine ran day and night.

Thank Goddess she had a mission, for bitterness was eating up the woman. The only thing the mercury mom hoped to recover was a settlement. She half-heartedly pursued dietary measures for her son, wondering aloud if supplements did any good at all. We regarded each other across a chasm of hope versus vengeful disillusionment.

The only biomedical approach the mercury mom pursued religiously was chelation. Her son had had several rounds, and Karen often brought out lab results showing all the mercury he'd "dumped." The chelators were actually rather like supplements, since most doctors were too afraid to prescribe them and most insurance didn't cover them.

I knew we needed to chelate Nina to remove any suspected mercury, but I held off. Kai shared my worries. Our daughter was the incarnation of "autistic with severe gut problems." Once the GFCF diet was in place, she went from the runs to Constipation City. We'd heard that if Nina's gut couldn't pass out the chelating compounds quickly enough, the toxic stuff would be re-absorbed as fresh mercury. Chelator supplements were also famous for making the yeast-beasts proliferate. Still, many parents considered the treatment the best thing they ever did for their afflicted child.

When I heard about a *transdermal* chelation compound called TD-DMPS, my intuition went into overdrive. DMPS was developed by the Soviets for detoxing miners and was said to target mercury. Transdermal DMPS was rubbed on the skin, bypassing the gut completely—now this was the ticket. Nina was seven when we began—almost at the upper age limit for reaping big results, according to Karen Carnes. Over several months, we rubbed the slightly smelly stuff onto every designated spot of thin skin where we had been told to rotate the applications.

Several things did fall into place for our daughter. We gauged a treatment, first and foremost, by Nina's quality and quantity of speech. DMPS gave her sentences meaning in place of sounds: the satisfaction of communication. Her repertoire and comprehension were limited, but we dared to believe she would someday be fully functional at the talking game.

Second, Nina began to play with toys. She still tapped and waved them, often unsure what to do with them and never doing it "right," but she was finally *interested* in toys. Until now, everything but books or the occasional light-up/beep-beep trinket had left her cold. Suddenly she took a shine to dolls and stuffed animals; she began to ride a tricycle, draw lines with sidewalk chalk outdoors, and climb over jungle gyms in the park. Her attitude was one of discovery. One day I ran in screaming to Kai, "She's playing in the sand box! She's playing in the sand box!" It was a treasure to watch her indifference and fears about normal-kid things fade away one by one.

And third, she slept better. Sometimes straight through the night. DMPS, how I loved you.

But did this mean she was mercury-poisoned? We ran toxic metals urine tests and never saw mercury in the results. Aluminum, cadmium, arsenic, lead—yes, too much. We saw the benefits but not the villain that the autism community longed to convict, that element named after the god with sandals winged.

Telltale poops

Rush hour was pushing hard in Kansas City as we drove home from our DAN doctor's office, chewing on bad news. Or was it good news? Finally, test results had showed Nina dumping more mercury than any other metal.

We'd squeezed into the doc's consulting room, devoid of toys for distraction. I knew Nina was claustrophobic and we didn't have long. But it didn't take long. Her lab results covered the small oval table between us. Pouring over the graphs, I wondered how many times the doctor had answered this question: "This is from her shots, right? Vaccines? And it's excessive, right?"

Since we were late in coming to these discoveries, I knew the skepticism out there—it came from school districts, from insurance companies, from people I thought were friends. But there was more; belief in immunizations dies hard.

"Has she eaten a lot of tuna lately?" our DAN man asked.

"No. We eat fish about once a week, or less. We never eat tuna, it has mercury in it," I said, like a dolt. Kai had the occasional tuna burger at a restaurant, but Nina and I had avoided the fish for years. "So…the mercury is from her immunizations, then?"

The elderly allergist who'd seen it all bobbed his head up and down.

No wonder the original lab analysis of a lock of hair showed little to no mercury. Unless the exposure was very recent, we learned, it would not show up in the hair of autistic children. Neurotypical, non-autistic children, on the other hand, might show a great deal of mercury in their hair samples—not because they were over-burdened with it, but because they were better excretors. They could get it out of their bodies. Unfortunately, those on the autism spectrum did not excrete the toxin as part of the normal detoxification process: it stayed tightly bound in their tissues.

Mercury. Mercury in Nina, and lots of it. *Someone has poisoned my baby.*

Mercury showed up in the poop, not in the urine or hair—we'd simply needed the right test. Now that there was proof, I was strangely calm.

But it was only the calm holding the eye of the storm. We were halfway home before emotions whirled me to the outer edges of the twister, and I was ready to flatten the responsible party.

It was simply not possible to avoid driving past the Boones' house, a tiny rancher two doors from a major thoroughfare. Each time I passed by, awash in resentment, I felt forced to look at the place. They'd dropped Nina (and us) for good. Now we all knew why.

If not the clueless Aidan, then Sandra the OB nurse and lactation expert surely knew something was not quite right with the infant

Nina. Maybe Sandra knew why her son and paramour were in a hurry to divest themselves of this baby—*because they too knew something was amiss*. Whether or not any of them were educated about autism, they surely knew Nina had quirks that might be abnormal and sought to unload her fast. Besides, Zeke and Carol had another child in tow, Carol's son from a previous marriage. He was a handful, showing signs of developmental delay in preschool.

The need for justice haunted me when it came to the Boones. No one should dispose of children simply because they were born under par. On the other hand, Aidan once said that the decision to relinquish Nina was the most responsible thing Zeke ever did. It seemed that everyone had benefited except Kai and I. Stating that fact plainly will sound cold to most ears, akin to saying we don't love her. Hear this: it takes daily contact with such a child to impart this rare mix of feeling screwed and yet at the same time blessed.

While many wait (and wait and wait) to adopt, false pretenses do not a serene adoption make. Sandra once stated, in all seriousness, that we didn't want to end up on *Oprah*, now did we? I stared at her. Our choice of options, open adoption, was commonplace. Was she referring to something I couldn't see? At the time, star-struck by Nina, I blinked and dismissed it. After all, Sandra could be such a drama queen.

But once talk spread of vaccinations as possible autism triggers and *epidemic* became a buzzword, pressure mounted within me to make the Boones pay. By twisted logic, I blamed them even more. Now it wasn't just their faulty genetic make-up—they had also exposed her to harmful vaccines. I felt that Sandra should have known better, but I overlooked the fact that health professionals are often the most conservative proponents of medicine-as-usual.

Kai was uncomfortable with such ruminations. I didn't want revenge so much as restitution, or at least a public shaming. He pointed out that there was no way we could prove prior knowledge of Nina's condition as an adoption by fraud. We couldn't legally press them to pay back any fraction of our mounting costs for her care and treatment. The public shaming would not be accomplished through the courts.

But there was more to Kai's distaste at my obsession with their wrongdoing. He himself was the product of a stepparent adoption, with an abusive stepfather who'd constantly complained about the money he wished he'd never spent on the boy. Kai couldn't bear the possibility of Nina feeling that we begrudged her a single thing. I loved him for that but continued to simmer, certain the Boones' karmic return would one day deliver.

I wasn't proud of myself for being filled to the brim with bile some days. I'd waited an extraordinarily long time to become a parent. Thanks to the Boones, I was a parent! But no thanks to them, we were a family torn apart.

It had been a long time since Kai called Nina his queen. His demeanor had gone from smitten to seriously distant. Perhaps, if he'd been the type to bond with loved ones in a crisis….but growing up he'd had absolutely no model for that. Instead of pressing him to do better, was I blaming the Boones for my lost last chance at a functional family? Although I knew there were spiritual tools available like radical forgiveness, the longing to see what goes around come around eventually won out.

The fall guy from Olympus

When people talk about vaccines and mercury, I often find myself thinking about Hermes, the Greek name for the Roman god Mercury.

On winged shoes he traversed lofty Olympus, the underworld, and the realms between—hence *quicksilver*, the common name for liquid mercury, that mysterious shiny line in the old thermometers, the mercurochrome stain for my ow-ies. Mercury is the metal, leaking from your dentist's handiwork, that finds its way into tissue and nerve. One drop kills the aquatic life in an entire lake. Quick silver indeed: fast moving and deadly.

But the Roman god Mercury was first named Hermes from the word *herm*, a pillar placed purposefully in simpler times to honor the fertility of the phallus. Long after the death of the old gods and the advent of the study of classical mythology, *Hg* became the abbreviation for quicksilver-mercury on the chart of chemical elements. But I feel sorry for Hermes, for in these steel-clad, ruined motherlands full of contaminated soil, water, and air, my skin crawls at what the word *mercury* conjures now. Mercury: the bane of our power plants, our medicine, the fillings in our sugared and staunched teeth. If Hermes still flies on winged feet, may he aid us in putting the careless and commercial use of his silver namesake back where it belongs.

The poison that Nina harbored in her cells was put there in the name of an innocent god. What a dirty trick.

Quicksilver: not for babies

The latest lab results got me thinking again about the Boones' genes. Maybe they had a genetic predisposition that weakened the ability to process toxic metals (a predisposition that might never have existed in our own biological child). Perhaps Nina's odds were further diminished because her birth mother grew up homeless, often hungry, and without medical care, while Zeke struggled with the world from a young age. But if even Nina wasn't launched with the greatest odds, what about all those kids from well-nourished, upper-crust families, the autistic children of brainy and robust parents? Such a widespread epidemic doesn't jibe with a simple genetic cause. Why would so many, in a relatively few short years, suddenly be so genetically susceptible?

I compared this situation with other worst-case scenarios. If nuclear winter should ever drape itself around the planet, how many people would have the genetics to withstand the radiation, the darkness, and the blight on all growing things? Most would die. Autism rates now stood at 1 per 88 children, and rising (or 1 in 43 boys) while 1 in 6 children worldwide were diagnosed with a developmental disorder. When will "many" become "most"?

Would these kids be perfectly healthy cherubs today, if not for vaccines laced with mercury preservatives? Could we draw the conclusion that mercury-free vaccines would spell the end to autism, developmental disorders, behavior problems?

The entire debate on mercury in childhood vaccines is masterfully laid out by David Kirby in *Evidence of Harm: A Medical Controversy*, an exhaustive study of the subject as of the year 2004. Kirby has authored countless articles on the topic since then. His resume is solid: an investigative journalist for many national magazines, he wrote regularly for the *New York Times* and *Newsday* and worked as a foreign correspondent for United Press International. He once served as a senior staff member of a well-known health research foundation.

Evidence of Harm was The Book that helped me come to grips with Nina's lab results. Not an easy read, but for me it was the essential read about autism for our times. When you're heading down the highway with bar-graph lines lunging out from a number of toxic metals (the longest line of all next to mercury), you need to know how to relate to the rest of the world. Kirby's book is largely the parents' story— no other players in the debate would talk to him—yet it also delves painstakingly into every nook and cranny of the issue. It's the story of moms—this time with the dads at their sides—as told by a journalist trained to dig for the truth.

A friend said, "I don't believe in conspiracy theories." End of discussion about the mercury in Nina's body. End of friendship, too; she found me tiresome. She didn't want to think about what's been done to children and other protected classes in the name of greed. If you don't think about it, perhaps it will never touch you.

I'd been there. When magic worked, I waxed evangelical about how each one of us was cause and effect in our lives. I steered clear of blaming the victim, but by the Goddess I swore I would never be one again. Magic would protect me from ever being duped—magic as double vision, keeping eyes on the everyday and on the spirit life. It worked, until it didn't. I couldn't keep a pregnancy, not even with the aid of spells, visits to Native American medicine men, trance, or prayer. I thought it was some kind of karmic re-pay until Nina lit up our days. Then she fell into a black hole, and I knew it wasn't my fault.

Or could I have "created her reality" to be normal and well? I was the one who took Nina in for her immunizations, wasn't I? I said *yes!* to the Boones' offer of a child to adopt, I believed their every word about her health, overlooked her quirks, and then sought to blame them and the faceless birth-mother when Nina didn't live up to my specs. Wasn't I now looking to blame the pharmaceutical companies, intent on raking in profits on vaccines, and government agencies who helped keep concerns about mercury-laden thimerosal under wraps? Were we, the parents of these poor autistic children, just grasping after someone to lynch—in the old days it was Tricky Dick Nixon, now it was Eli Lilly? Were we exhibiting nothing more than grief-crazed group-think, a mob out for blood and screaming at the corporate wall?

Drug 'em if you can't spank 'em no more

Let me see if I've got this right. First, we compound ever more vaccines to wipe out disease, using risky ingredients to spread the practice far and wide—cheaply. When kids get meaner, less social, or can't learn, we make new drugs to make them behave. That way, you catch them coming and going.

Drugging children has replaced corporal punishment: the father's belt on the butt, the swats from the principal, the open-handed slaps in the face once favored by mothers and nuns. Abusive, of course, so what about a teeny pill? Far more socially acceptable. Yet this chemical spanking can scar a child for life.

As a scruffy runaway looking for the next high, I was convinced that I was entitled to nonstop pleasure, that I hurt no one with my psychedelic voyages, that the green of homegrown weed was proof that we were natural, hence Good. Back in those days, when the position of heir to the Wohler Madness was up for grabs, when my reckless teenaged hunger met up with the Habitat's official neglect, I learned just what pharmaceuticals could do. My solitary, voluntary brush with Thorazine in 1969 was an episode I specifically declined to repeat, despite my ongoing teenage quest for new and better highs. Thorazine made me afraid in ways that no "tribal" drug ever had.

The irony that *they* would dare to cure a drug problem with *their* drugs was not lost on our tribe, whether inside the hospital or out. The hospital staff, from the greater powers in the front office down to the lowly aides, saw it this way: *they* had medicine, while we had only entrepreneurs—dealers who paid no taxes. The drugs handed out by sedate nurses on med-line were supposed to make me well, while sneaky drugs jeopardized my sanity. *They* had research to back up which side they chose to stand on.

But how did Pharma convince the world it had the only pure stuff in the first place? From the days of the Inquisition to the asylum to the chemical straightjacket, it's all about social control (as the B-brothers once ranted). Plus an added effort that sealed the deal: marketing.

That's how Pharma got Sam. How did he survive on their wares for two decades and counting? I guess it depends on your definition of survival. I was still looking for some answer that would spring Sam free when I read *Mad in America: Bad Science, Bad Medicine, and the Enduring Mistreatment of the Mentally Ill* by Robert Whitaker. What I found was a penetrating history of the mental health profession that described the rise of the first antipsychotic drug: chlorpromazine, better known by its trade name, Thorazine. A super-high dose was Sam's mainstay until the new "atypical" antipsychotics hit the market. Since Thorazine had shaped so much of his adult life—and nearly scared me, literally, to death—I raced with hunger, then horror, through Whitaker's account.

I learned that Thorazine hailed from a group of compounds first used to make synthetic dyes, then insecticides. When someone noticed that the substance curtailed locomotion in mammals without putting them to sleep, it was tried as an anesthesia. Thorazine gained a reputation for inducing a waking hibernation, a supreme detachment and indifference. Soon, psychiatrists were using the new drug to calm patients in rowdy madhouses across the United States.

But peace for the mental health staff came with a price for the patients. Symptoms of Parkinson's disease and encephalitis lethargica, also known as sleeping sickness, burgeoned. Since at first no one pretended that Thorazine was a cure, some rather prominent voices protested. But what happened next, Whitaker reveals, was far more about money than healing.

The more I read, the more proud I grew of my father's rebel stance against his family's pressure to become a doctor. The year that young Robert Elton dreamed of teaching literature at Harvard, legislation toppled the American Medical Association's position as watchdog over the drug companies. Now doctors became the sole conduit for dispensing most drugs. Pharma mobilized to court and "educate" physicians about their products, and a love affair between the two camps was born. Had my dad become a physician, what would he have done? Would he have followed the money or seen the folly of Pharma's scheme?

Whitaker notes that the drug companies could get easier FDA approval and charge higher prices in the U.S. than in other countries. With doctors in their corner, they needed only to convince politicians—and the public. Thus began the campaign to switch Thorazine's image from chemical lobotomy to miracle cure, using articles in popular magazines from writers highly paid by Pharma to do their dirty work.

Medical journals fared no better. Pharmaceutical companies ghostwrote many of the positive articles that supposedly came from scientific minds, while references to dangerous side effects were deleted.

After that revelation I had to set aside Whitaker's text for awhile. Don't tell the daughter of English teachers that writers of all people—that feisty, independent lot—were paid to say what industry told them to!

But read on I finally did, and Whitaker showed how writers weren't the only smart people taken in. Pharma's marketing machine worked on state legislators to get more money for research, in the interest of emptying out the mental hospitals through use of the wonder drug, Thorazine. In the early 1960's, when President John Kennedy promoted a new vision of community health supported by plentiful neighborhood clinics, Thorazine was the antipsychotic vehicle to enable this new Enlightenment.

Is there a parallel story with thimerosal, the mercury-containing preservative in vaccines? Since the public hardly knew it was there until recently, no sell job was required if all could be kept under wraps. Babies can only protest with their cries.

There is speculation that academics and bureaucrats in government agencies may have been asleep at the wheel when it came to adding up thimerosal's dangerous numbers. But as more parents retained counsel, attorneys uncovered that Eli Lilly, the makers of thimerosal, had cloaked its danger since 1930.

Camelot comes riding

When I was a girl attending Catholic school amidst nuns, lay teachers, and students in uniform, there was no one closer to God the Father than the Kennedys. When JFK was elected to the presidency, the elementary students played like monkeys the next day at recess, screaming like banshees and running like wildfire all over the grounds. We were high on our parents' glee: *a Catholic, finally, at the helm of our country!* But for most people the Beautiful Family was just that: attractive, charmed and, of course, super-smart. So when the King of Camelot was shot down, the schoolchildren immediately were sent home, but we did more: we crowded into churches and wept. Hard.

I didn't want to pray. Later, as a young hippie, when I heard they had shot his brother, the next heir to Camelot, I wanted someone to pay—and embraced the radical rhetoric of revolution. Now a parent of a child with autism, I understand waiting for a long time to be heard by the right people. But finally a knight of Camelot—nephew of the fallen king, son of the fallen presumed heir—is listening.

Robert Kennedy, Jr. publicly shared his journey from skeptic to concerned environmentalist after he had reviewed drug companies' efforts to maintain silence about thimerosal. An attorney for the Natural Resources Defense Council, this knight from Camelot was concerned about many things. Like the secret meeting focused on how to downplay thimerosal, convened by the CDC at an isolated retreat center and attended by representatives from every major drug company, where information was "embargoed"—no photocopies allowed, no papers taken off the grounds. Or the exhaustive list of studies that Eli Lilly ignored, concerning the susceptibility of primates to brain damage from thimerosal. Independent researchers denied access to a database paid for with taxpayer money. A government directive to the Institute of Medicine to whitewash the link between autism and thimerosal. Sir Kennedy concluded that this was "a moral crisis that must be addressed."

Camelot may or may not be an outdated notion, but at least one descendant cared. Maybe we can reverse the damage that occurred when the knight's uncle inadvertently gave Pharma the right to damage minds with his plan for "community mental health." But I can't help wondering: Is it enough? Is this all about vaccines? Am I, when it comes to Nina, jumping to conclusions—clutching her lab results because it's a real piece of paper, it's scientific, it's all I have?

Beyond vaccines

Besides mercury in vaccines, it comes to us in the air from coal-fired plants, in fish that could have replaced cow as healthful nourishment, in countless over-the-counter products we buy everyday. But other scientific findings crowd at me like so many clamoring voices, insisting mercury is not the only contaminant that assails children and sensitive body-minds. Food dyes can provoke uncontrollable rage and weeping fits. Pesticides, industrial solvents, and chlorinated brews with unattractive names may explain why Johnny brings guns to school. Hormone-disrupters set off early puberty—thus girls under the age of ten dress like hookers, and we blame *them* as insatiable consumers. But there is no meaner toxin than mercury. If you have a child with autism, all you want to do is dig out the one root and then rest.

Now that autism rates are climbing in other countries, will there even be a chance to rest? How many more toe-walking, hand-flapping, obsessive-compulsive, anxiety-driven, food-sensitive, chemical-burdened, metabolism-disordered children will be treated with operant conditioning ("Like dog training!" says Kai) so that parents get some semblance of control? If you don't have a child like this, someone in your extended family probably does, or one lives in your neighborhood. There is one or more in your child's classroom, there is a child at church. Or maybe you see autism in the news now and again. Maybe you were one of those complaining about the hype over autism in *USA Today*. (Gee, I'm sorry—don't want to hear about autism? Fine. Until you love some child who has it. Then I will dry your tears, too.)

But the mercury moms and dads know that there is a huge gap between issues bandied about in the press, and a real grasp of vaccines as dangerous. They know they are fighting uphill when they blow the whistle loudly in order to make the shots safe. Like me, no one wants to give a child over to disease. I hate being thrust between the lesser of two evils; I hate the possibility that the immunizations supposed to save my child from epidemics may have created the saddest epidemic of all.

Okay, I'm angry. But I might be more settled if I could say with one hundred percent conviction what caused Nina's autism. Though mercury is a mighty toxic load, what about the thousands of other unstudied chemicals in use? That boatload of potentially toxic items that no one's ever bothered to fully assess for danger raises the possibility that any one of them—or several in combination—could deliver an autistic wham. What if Nina's birth mother, homeless and hungry, was a pregnant migrant worker blasted by pesticides from a low-flying prop-plane? Or what if the family, living in their car, had parked near a hazardous waste site? Hermes' namesake could only make matters worse. Was Nina autistic before she ever entered our home, flapping her fists at the Boones' parakeet, staring into bright lights, preferring her bottle alone, inspecting rattles but never shaking them? There was mercury aplenty coursing through her then. Things took a turn for the worst after the MMR—or did we just notice the unmet milestones as she grew older?

The inability to pin down the first—or at least major—cause rips at my heart like a junkyard dog. Because, like anyone helplessly hoping, I need at least this one point of closure.

Chapter 16
WHEN FAMILY WON'T LISTEN

One year after Pfeiffer, Nina was still seizure-free. We considered it a miracle, and I couldn't help but think about the possibilities for Ben's boys, my nephews. Throughout the adoption process, there had been little information available about their health legacy. As in Nina's case, one could assume there was some affliction in the birth family's tree. In Cambodia, as in most of Southeast Asia, the government handles adoptions, and cultural mores unfortunately dictate silence when the father is unknown. All the more reason, in my opinion, to do some testing in case there were *physiological* roots to the boys' supposedly psychological disorders.

When I tried to discuss alternative treatments with my brother Ben, he was adamant that Paul and Pete, his "ADHD poster children," must stay on drugs—or, as he preferred to call it, "stimulant therapy." Couldn't he see Nina was better? She was making real sentences and her long fits of frustration were gone. It was as I'd told Kai: through her newfound sense of *presence*, Nina had finally joined our family.

But she was not yet "fully recovered," as Ben pointed out. He suggested that, as far as the seizures went, maybe Nina just "grew out of 'em."

When I described the zinc-copper theory, gluten and dairy sensitivity, and high histamine, my younger brother listened politely. But as soon as I mentioned the potential for his own sons, he shot me the squint-eye. I could see the Keep Out sign on the gate.

Days later, Ben gathered up the scoffings of Internet pundits who live to debunk medical myths and forwarded them to me. We took part in some brother-sister sparring, pitting one set of research and news articles against another. I was the one who finally backed off. Painful as it was to witness my nephews medicated into an unproductive trance, in the end it was the cold fury of their parents toward alternative treatments that made me shelve a lost cause.

My brother never considered ADHD part of the "autism spectrum." The boys were not *that*, just less-fortunates from the Third World. (Not that they spoke of Cambodia to the boys; Cambodia was irrelevant.) This was during a time when ADHD was becoming accepted parlance for kids who could barely help it, what with TV and the breakdown of the family.

Medicating the boys with Ritalin—then Adderall, then Concerta—took place during a power shift between husband and wife. Pam was making a career leap just as Ben severed all professional ties to become a stay-at-home dad. The needs of the two hyperactive half-brothers necessitated that one parent sacrifice a life. How well I understood.

Our kids can't help being who they are. Society says it doesn't want anyone to hide "special" kids from view anymore. So the likes of Benny and I must hide instead. Who is being protected from whom here? Either we chafe when people exalt us as "special needs parents," or we fume because they don't acknowledge our stressed and stranded situation.

Or we resent the hell out of *them* for having a life that must be better than ours. We resent the extra investment of time, the intensity of labor. Since our children are adopted, we come off looking like saints. But with one Wohler ancestor kept alive in the annals of the history of chemistry, with the pile-up of our father's awards and publications standing in stark contrast to the lost promise of Sam's brain, our setbacks are painfully manifest. Ben and I had set the family name backwards by several unnatural steps. Despite everything that our kids will never grasp about us, what they sense, on some inchoate but enduring level, is our gut feeling that they are not the ones who failed. We did.

Ben is vigilant with his sons whenever the family gathers in private or public. Likewise, we're hot on Nina's trail. At the slightest hint of a turned back, she will sneak into chocolate, not always diet-approved. Or break someone's cherished memento. Or run off down the road. The boys come with stories of dangerous performances that they thought were good clean fun, stories that go beyond "boys will be boys" or "they're a handful." Tension has remodeled my brother's face into that of a prison guard working long shifts. Am I like that with Nina?

She is beautiful and female—and white. If the world seems more forgiving of her antics than those of two dark-skinned boys from Cambodia (especially ones who live in Texas), then my brother, the family expert on appearing normal, keeps hyper-vigilant for a reason. He must publicly show that he sides with White Normal Texas in expecting transgressions and being poised to deal with them.

Even at a young age Ben displayed the urge—the one that afflicted all but Narcissus and me—toward self-restriction. Hold back, so no one is offended. Then he found car culture, where it's all-American to be obsessed with chrome and lube and the friendships come with the territory. Ben was the lost boy in a family he couldn't figure out.

As an adoring younger sibling, Benny felt I could do no wrong. Yet in those days I increasingly closed out the little brother who always wanted to come into my room, listen to my music, be with my friends. Everybody knew little brothers are a pain to teenage girls and no one reprimanded me. The hurt look on his face was easily blocked out. I had troubles of my own, and he was my parents' problem to attend to.

Benny carved his own niche, although at what price there is no way to know. He is the escapee from our strangeness. He turned his back on the bookish stuff to hunker down with the locals, and passed. Am I the only one who sees it in his eyes still, the sign flickering there that reads, "Lost boy! Lost boy! Somebody please come find me!"?

Once, I tried to tell my brother that I was sorry for my self-absorption when we were growing up. Ben received my confession with an embarrassed "don't worry about it," but his eyes, for one instant, were wet.

How envious I was that, despite a diagnosis and a special education classroom, Paul and Pete could play soccer and basketball and hold their own at a video arcade. Except for their drug fuzz (and few friends who visit their house), they seemed so normal compared to Nina. They are fun-loving boys who, when not over-medicated, are drawn to people. Computers are taking over but each still has a ready smile for those who look past the color of their skin. Nina they find amusing. I get irritated at their open sniggering, but I suppose they've received the same in spades. When it comes to them and me, we move like magnets to one another. "Aunt Sue" is music to my ears. Do they sense my desire to help them?

One time the whole crew came to visit our place. Down at the creek, I tried to show the boys fossils, slate, and crawdads. Each offering held them for only a split-second of attention before they charged unceremoniously onward. I was simply pleased to have them in my sacred spot, but Ben wanted to see some awe, curiosity, or fellow feeling from the two. His open contempt for them was so reminiscent our father. During our stroll he was quick with threats at the slightest acceleration of their energy. My brother would not listen to friendly suggestions that he lighten up. "You don't know," he warned, "what they can get into."

What are your days worth when you must police each mood and every movement of another human being? What is it like to be the other on such a leash, braided out of love and fear?

The heartbreak for me is that, although the Pfeiffer Center didn't bring Nina—poof!—back into normalcy, it might have landed Paul and Pete there. The boys' mania for dairy foods is legendary; they are fed ice cream for breakfast. The additives they ingest in various snack foods are as routine as the sun rising through their Hot Wheels curtains. Prescription lotion is needed for their skin, so painfully dry. Omega-3 fish oils could have soothed that leather and sharpened their wits. But when I mused to Benny about the healthier diet in the boys' native country, he gawked at me like a redneck stuck in the company of a kook.

A sister not credible

Most of us are trained to seek authorities outside the bounds of family, someone whose professionalism hides fault and makes for an easy leap of faith. Ben's tendency toward frequent headaches inspired no interest in what I'd discovered about mine. There was too much history to step around. To define oneself is to separate, says the culture.

My stay at the Habitat, although to this day never referenced by Ben, shot down my credibility.

In 1968 my self-designated tribe and I were given the biggest guns in Pharma's arsenal, despite the fact that adolescent brains and bodies were still finding their way through critical growth stages. (It was during this time that I began having migraines, passed off as menstrual troubles.) And what of the fragility of elderhood? If nutrients had been handed out instead of drugs in the "med lines" of the mental hospitals, would my grandmother still have tried to strangle herself with the belt of a terrycloth robe? Would I have terrified my family by running away from home? Would I have flinched at an incoming volleyball? Over and over, I was forced to overhaul my assessment of the Great Plains Mental Health Habitat experience. *What if the Inquisitors were just as toxic in their body-minds as I was?* It was this thought that eventually broke the hold of that hatred I'd taken away from the whole experience.

I often ask myself why I must painfully witness this repeat of social control exercised on younger and younger children—including those I am related to. I'd give anything to understand those who shun explanations of how body toxins affect behavior, who opt instead for years of ineffective therapies and a life of stigma. I'll wager that Ben is influenced more by his personal past than by research. He needs to dampen the antics of Pete and Paul so he won't risk anything resembling that time when his big sister—or grandmother Agnes—was out-of-control.

At least Ben has never said out loud, *Nina needs medication!* He must feel he's taken the high road, going one better than my entreaties to let Pete and Paul try life drug-free. But his feelings are obvious in the way that he and his wife ignore Nina. If she is loud, they are as disapproving as any stranger. If food goes flying, I can almost hear my brother's thoughts: *Would an SSRI help? One of the new atypicals?* When we can't calm her and she must flee or be removed, sympathy is never the response. *She's such a mess. You should do **anything** to get her to behave.*

Ben was still in elementary school when I disappeared for one month in Denver as the incorrigible runaway, then spent six months more at a mental hospital. My little brother suffered horribly with anxious stomachaches during that time. Running away from home was a major betrayal on the part of his sister. What might it have to do with him? Then she was put in a place that proved she was somehow sick—in her mind, they said. I'd lost him forever, and now I couldn't even help his lost boys.

Sam's last stand

It was pouring and blowing cold rain as I drove the rental car to the Pfeiffer Treatment Center. Sam trembled in his thin, shapeless overcoat and cranked the heater insufferably high. As soon as we entered the building, he high-tailed it back outside for one more smoke. The awning was pitifully short, and the elements had their way with my older brother as he sucked at the small fire to steady his nerves.

I checked in with the receptionist and watched Sam huddle before the plate glass. I remembered the moment when, months ago, I'd first presented the idea of coming here. We were at his favorite diner, the kind of place that forever postpones much-needed remodeling (don't look at the mangy carpet, watch out for tables with one leg too short). Nonetheless, it was something of a coup to even get him out of the house. Not because he was afraid to mix in public (as long as the places were known), but because his girlfriend kept close tabs on him. She didn't go out much and, frankly, she found my ideas dangerous. She didn't know what I was up to this time, and I'd planned it that way.

At the diner I told Sam what the Pfeiffer clinic had done for Nina. I was stepping gingerly, ready to take a roundabout approach: build a case, then deal with denial and excuses and let it wait for a better day, hopefully soon. Sam was aging fast. Long gone were the days he was actively advocating for the rights of fellow consumers. Long gone were the therapy appointments, trying this or that method. Sam cooked and cleaned and waited on a girlfriend who periodically alienated their one friend, leaving Sam alone with her for weeks at a time. With his white Santa Claus beard, where food often fell and remained, and fingernails like long claws, his visage was sculpted into a look of perpetual alarm. The muscle spasms and tics were called tardive dyskinesia—a common side effect of many psychiatric drugs.

Ironically, my brother no longer heard voices nor wanted to avoid people—yet now he thoroughly looked the part of someone bearing the paranoiac's burden. Anti-psychotic drugs gave him a dragging limp, a waxen stare, saliva that slipped uncontrollably from the sides of his mouth. Ill-fitting, fashion-defying clothes—all of it was just Sam, but it seemed almost macabre now that his frame was hunched and emaciated, subject to odd jerks at odd times. Sam didn't inhabit this body. He simply bore it as best he could.

Some would say that the drugs finally worked, controlling his paranoia and keeping him on track for the rest of his days. He was still on Haldol, had participated in clinical trials for Seroquel and took a high dose. When his girlfriend convinced their mutual shrink that Sam was depressed, Lexipro was lobbed in for good measure. On top of that were a dozen assorted pharmaceuticals for high blood pressure, arthritis, and other complaints of midlife. This was the best his doctors could do over the decades to get a semblance of normal behavior. I preferred to believe that it was love that gave Sam his lifeline. His girlfriend's disability was far more problematic than his, and he rallied—as he put it—"to dote on her."

I'd practiced unraveling my spiel. The Pfeiffer clinic had a fund for the indigent, and we could get Sam covered by it. My brother finished his third Coke in less than five minutes, and broke in. "When can we go?"

As I paid the bill, we shared a festive moment. We hadn't done anything together like this in—actually, well, *ever*.

On the flight to Chicago, Sam enjoyed the ride like a child. He was sanguine about taking off his shoes in the security line and seemed to fear nothing. It had been so long since he'd seen this much adventure that he imbibed and stored its power for later, for that long stretch of cigarettes, television, and living at the girlfriend's beck and call.

Nicotine fix complete, Sam pulled his coat tighter against the Windy City and ground the filter onto wet pavement. My smile, as he walked in, tried to impart bravery as I dared to think that his troubles might end. I believed that this clinic and its colleagues of like mind were poised to cure autism. They'd reached to the root of why our most heinous murderers were prompted to kill. But schizophrenia was their real forte, dating to the days when Carl Pfeiffer himself still lived. Fixing Sam should be a slam-dunk.

The nurse called for Sam, and together we made the circuit of the various tests—a door here, another there. He hadn't been able to afford glasses in a long time and needed help filling out the forms. The halls were still adorned with the impressive storyboards detailing the Center's research on serial killers. I read it all again.

Carl Pfeiffer's major contribution to healing schizophrenia was his discovery of pyroluria, a Vitamin B-6 and zinc deficiency. A nurse showed us the telltale white spots on Sam's overgrown fingernails and assured us that his compounded supplements would include zinc. I wondered if Sam was as copper-toxic as Nina and, if so, whether he'd been like that as a teenager when everything started to go awry for him.

I was thrilled when the staff acknowledged my brother's background in physics and chemistry. One even said, "Maybe you'll be able to help us someday," and Sam beamed. I noticed he had several teeth missing, and made a silent note to look into charities that cover dental work. As with Nina's intake, no prognosis was ventured until the labs were available to point the way.

The supplements arrived. Sam's case manager was supportive and enthusiastic, his psychiatrist skeptical but tolerant. The case manager loaded the huge compounded pills into Sam's daily med box. Hopes were high.

The clearing

I called every other day to check on my brother. After ten days of Sam on the supplements, hopes rose even higher.

Sam, before and during our travels to the Pfeiffer clinic, was monosyllabic; he struggled for words, staring hard at you so he could track. I had to repeat things, realizing that normal speech whizzed by him too fast. His slurred speech reminded me of someone fighting off sleep, with the nuances of conversation well out of reach. It was hard to spend much time together when silence only lengthened the shadow between us.

On the tenth day after our trip to Pfeiffer, I called my brother again. "So? How's this working out for you overall?" I asked.

"Pretty good, pretty good. I feel a strength and clarity I haven't felt in years."

A strength and clarity I haven't felt in years. The phrasing, the articulation, and the appropriate emotional tone: it felt like a miracle. It was as if Nina had one day awakened and said, "Hi Mom, what's for breakfast?"

I quoted Sam many times over the course of what unfolded next. That sentence became a herald, a poem, a manifesto whose exact words I will never forget. On the nutrient path, when family listens and you can help, there is no greater relief. I made a point to replay it often in my head. *A strength and clarity I haven't felt in years.*

During this upswing, another event revealed even more about emergence than Sam's renewed vocabulary. When the simple but portentous event occurred, I thought, *Now, we're really getting somewhere!*

My brother retained an apartment in the same complex as his girlfriend, frequently retreating there when she threw him out after a fight. She would call him minutes or hours later, and he'd dutifully cross the complex and knock on her door. Shortly after the strength and clarity of past years revived him, they'd had another tiff over nothing. Sam was berated and verbally abused as before, but his time *he* left voluntarily for his own apartment. "She's not going to treat me like that anymore!" he said with conviction in his voice when I phoned.

I felt on top of the world. The real Sam was back.

But by the third week, Sam was fatigued and frantic. He found it hard to walk. He couldn't keep his eyes open, and his girlfriend was upset that he was unable to wait on her. What was going on?

Pfeiffer said the supplements were working. Decrease the Seroquel.

Sam's psychiatrist at the mental health center was firm: *nothing doing.*

Obscuring the obvious

If only my brother had had David Moyer to guide his way.

Moyer, a former military therapist, cured his teenage son of severe bipolar disorder with nutrients. He tells the story in his book, *Too Good to Be True? Nutrients Quiet the Unquiet Brain.*

When Moyer's son was institutionalized, the boy began developing Parkinsonian symptoms. Moyer and his wife snuck in supplements, disguised in a bag of peanuts and candy. Probably due to Moyer's social-worker profession, the hospital relented when he pressed them to lower his son's dose of Zyprexa. The symptoms stopped. Moyer figured out that the supplements had increased the potency of the medication.

Sam could barely handle his Seroquel as it was. He complained of sleeping seventeen hours a day. Clearly, the Pfeiffer change for the better came sooner than anyone had anticipated. I'd believed Sam's psychiatrist when she said she was on board. I hadn't anticipated how she would react if the supplements worked fast.

The mental health center sent him to a general practice M.D., thinking the answer might be a liver problem. I spoke to the doctor personally. There was nothing wrong with Sam's liver, he said. There was nothing wrong with Sam at all, aside from his psych issues and bothersome arthritis.

I tried next to convince Dr. Botchkin, Sam's psychiatrist, to back down the Seroquel and let Sam get the full benefit of the Pfeiffer protocol. She stopped taking my calls.

They were wasting time, stalling, while Sam was getting worse—and more freaked out.

I arranged a conference call between Dr. Botchkin and Dr. Devera, a Pfeiffer psychiatrist and veteran of a long administrative career in the Illinois mental health system. He was in his "second career," post retirement, and enthusiastic about what nutrition could do for the mentally ill. Working within "the system," Dr. Devera had seen it all, clearly topping Sam's shrink in experience. He explained to her why it was time now, right now, to slowly titrate down Sam's meds so the vitamins and supplements could have their maximum effect.

I could tell that this was going to be a hard sell. Dr. Botchkin sat like a fortress, as closed as a double agent full of secrets. She inhabited her chair like a mountain practiced in making its surface impenetrable.

When she glanced my way, she allowed a barely concealed distaste to show through, for she had so many more important things to do than haggle about vitamins with a demanding family member.

Dr. Botchkin reminded us that she intended to wait a full six months before she would consider lightening up the big guns' hold on Sam. We pointed out that her patient's body-mind necessitated a quicker timetable. But for this matron, weighed down no doubt by bureaucracy's daily grind, it was imperative to win. Her explanation was that she didn't want to do anything to hurt Sam. As if the tics, salivating, slurred words, and Haldol's "grinding sound" in his head were helping him!

The stalling dragged on. Now not even Sam's case manager would return my calls. Sam was beside himself; his girlfriend was livid. She made it her mission to convince him of the danger of Pfeiffer's protocol. Finally, pressed to the wall by the veiled threats of the mental health system—*Do you want us to cut your case management? Your transportation? Food pantries?*—Sam's last defensive words were, "I guess the vitamins don't work for me."

Too much was at stake. Sam was afraid. He'd been a ward of the system's beneficence too long. I tried to find another psychiatrist to take over Sam's case. The problem was, my indigent brother needed to use Medicaid. In all of the Kansas City area, I could not match enthusiasm for nutrient therapy with this necessary financial restriction.

I recalled the little inspirational book on courage I gave him before we went to Pfeiffer. It was about the Hindu goddess Kali—not the Durga form with serene face that I looked at daily, but she of the fearsome visage who is so easily misunderstood. Though She dances on the body of Her consort wearing a necklace of bloody skulls, brandishing knives and swords and destroying that which is outworn, She is a most beloved goddess in Her culture. For it's understood that in order to create we must destroy, that change is inevitable and natural and involves the pain of severance at times. I suggested to Sam that he needed courage to sever from what may have been comfortably known. I showed him the mudra, or hand position, that Kali makes to Her worshippers: one hand raised as if in greeting, palm facing straight outward. *Fear not.*

But Sam lacked the stamina for butting heads, and used up all his courage walking inside the Pfeiffer Center's front door. Neither a rebel nor, for all his enthusiasm about science, a free thinker, he'd always followed the directives of authorities. How could he start to think now with clarity? The life of chemical straightjacketing left no foundation on which to build.

No matter how I tried to get around her, Dr. Botchkin would not be moved. Up in Illinois, there was little that Dr. Devera, the experienced consultant for Pfeiffer, could do. My mother began to complain about his hefty hourly fee.

Pharma had won. One more potentially brilliant physicist lost to the world. One more bonus pack of brain power dismantled by the mental health system.

❋ ❋ ❋

I didn't want to admit, it but I missed my dad. At the time Sam and I flew to Pfeiffer, he hadn't been dead a year. Alive and at the helm, he might have made Dr. Botchkin see the light—when it came to bullying bureaucrats, he always rose to the occasion. Now, instead, our mother was still adjusting to widowhood. Her husband had handled everything, and she was not the sort to take on the likes of a busy psychiatrist, the director of an entire county treatment center.

Would my father have scoffed at the vitamins, too? I couldn't imagine it. He'd tried to reason with Ben, advising against putting the boys on drugs, but of course Benny exercised the upper hand as parent—or, more to the point, Ben complied with Pam's upper hand. Would my father have risen to save Sam, or would he have rendered this sacrifice to the Wohler Madness?

Since I was "just a mom" (and "only a sibling" to the patient at that), I failed to wield the authority that Robert Elton could have invoked. I could not be him, even when it was most called for. I accepted it when Dr. Botchkin pulled the plug on our hopes, but somehow I felt the failure was mine.

Sam was back to square one. Dr. Botchkin raised his dose of Seroquel, just for spite. My brother was mad at me, and running a number on himself that the Pfeiffer experiment had hurt him. His girlfriend was haughty; feeling vindicated, she joined in the blame-heaping. Kai, who had provided the airfare and cash for the trip, was peeved along with the rest when Sam quit taking the Pfeiffer supplements. Our mother wouldn't say who she believed. Up in Chicago, at the end of their charity for the likes of Sam, the Pfeiffer Clinic closed his file.

Chapter 17
ANSWERING FOR THE ANCESTOR

Even though chemists as a group are not noted for their great beauty, Friedrich Wohler was an outstandingly homely man.

Surely this call depends on the eye of the beholder? An online history of chemistry is equally rude, stating that Wohler resembled a cross between Abraham Lincoln, the Supremes, and a horse. Yet any photograph of the man makes it hard to miss that hair: what lift, what a sweep of curls! The wild locks defy German stereotypes of strict compliance and Aryan might. If we inherited nothing else, it was the tendency toward thick hair.

In a portrait of the scientist as a young man, Wohler gazes out over a cravat that looks like a rag around his columnar neck. He's bony and angular like I was in my anorectic youth. Like me, young Friedrich went all over the great outdoors. Like Sam, he built a chemistry lab in his father's house.

One historian of chemistry noted "that passionate love of nature which was so strikingly exhibited in the man.... He had, moreover, to thank his father for that love of physical exercise and passion for outdoor life." Friedrich's father ran the stables at a royal household, serving as both veterinarian and horse trader. He made sure his son was taught sketching "and otherwise educated in that perception of natural beauty." It felt good to know that Wohler began comfortably in the bosom of Mother Earth and the arts.

Reading about Wohler's apparently functional yet supportive family, it's hard to trust that he's really one of us. The Wohlers didn't badger young Friedrich to follow anyone's footsteps, nor did they snuff out the flame with indifference or envy. His self-taught knowledge of chemistry enabled him to skip university lectures on the subject. With a mind ripe for formal training, it was agreed he should study abroad with older, more gifted individuals.

So much for chips off the old block. He was industrious, noticed, and apparently chafed against no restraints.

Yet I struggle to get around stereotypes of his times. Victorians: the stuffy, the corseted, the repressed. Fainting hysterical women, children working fingers to the bone in factories both unsafe and unhealthy. Freud. Asylums full of women who protested the rule of husbands, fathers, church.

Contrast that to the happy Wohler, traipsing through nature, pursuing knowledge without a hitch. Numerous reports of his sanguine character kept me asking at what point, exactly, did our genes go wrong? How can I relate to this even-tempered explorer, prolific without vainglory or heart attacks, pursuing his passion among like-minded friends? Where's the narcissism, the fits of rage, the bitter rivals, the inner conflicts to stall his steps?

I knew that one Wohler pitfall was to be paralyzed by loss. But even after his first wife took ill and died, Friedrich worked the grief out of himself. Friend Liebig brought him over to his lab and the two remained busy, side by side, until Friedrich recovered. Onward he worked and worked, living to the age of eighty-two. Spending forty-six years at the University of Gottingen, where Benjamin Franklin studied as a young man, he made the school famous for chemistry. He sired four more children with a second wife—did he ever see them while garnering medals and accolades, playing with fire, and living to tell packed lecture halls about it? Was he even expected to spend time with his children? I'm reaching here, trying to find a flaw, because what I really want to know is this: where *was* the Wohler Madness back then?

How could we, less than a hundred years later, have deteriorated from the lofty standard he set? Why couldn't we have inherited a slice of that drive and inspiration—or was my father the last one skirting close? Why have subsequent generations produced their share of modern-day lepers, mad hatters, loony slackers, all a drain on a family's pride and resources?

Until Nina made me rethink these questions, the genius-nutcase dichotomy in our genetic line was all right with me. We were willing to risk madness if it meant genius might be forthcoming at the hidden roulette wheel of our fates. In the old days, I simply concluded that Friedrich Wohler had lucked out—he could have easily been one of the fallen.

Separating spirit from nature

I doubt Wohler imagined what he was setting in motion. There were enough lands unexplored on the globe to make foreseeing its poisoning, dangerous warming, and the extinction of entire species a stretch for the rational mind. He wasn't the only thinker of his time who now appears to us as, well, blithe. Working with a web of men who felt they were onto something big, who were driven to synthesize, synthesize, synthesize. Consciously trying to rob Life itself of glory? Or smitten with a fever for inquiry? Besides, he was no Galileo; he wasn't up against the Church, so it was all right to play demigod.

He was 28 years old when he synthesized the first organic compound, urea, completely by accident.

The theories of Vitalism were still in place. *This is organic*—sugar, olive oil, anything which when subject to fire will smoke, fume, or char. *This is inorganic*: water, salt, and the like. That was final, and who knows if Friedrich ever doubted it. He approached the lab unsuspecting on that day, ready to pursue those puzzling white crystals that formed whenever he mixed cyanic acid and ammonium. Not to challenge the known rules of life itself.

In a passage I find chilling, Wohler foretells the future.

The philosophy of chemistry will conclude from this work that it must be held not only as probable but [as] certain that all organic substances, insofar as they no longer belong to the organism, will be prepared in the laboratory. Sugar, salicin, morphine will be produced artificially. It is true that the route to these end products is not yet clear to us, because the intermediaries from which these materials develop are still unknown, but we shall learn to know them.

How can I answer for him—was he thoroughly amoral, or should he be forgiven for his blindness to the dangers? Personally loving Nature, professionally out to fabricate everything natural inside the lab, as if to outdo the mystery of Creation itself. What a thrill—to do what The Goddess does! How tempting, how can one turn it down? And why assume it would bring your descendants anything but pleasure and ease?

After my Habitat stay and the fall of Sam the Brain, I learned to accept that the family disease in my generation meant a slide from Friedrich Wohler's capabilities into the rubble of under-achievement. I spent decades believing we were lazy or crazy, until Nina blew the lid off this self-flagellation. Once her example led me down the nutrient path into a profound clearing of mind, our family's great lethargy, self-restriction, and paranoid fantasies started to appear less like the Wohler Madness and more like a toxic load.

Whose side would Wohler be on now? I think about how he appeared in my gathering of guides by the river—why was he so focused on the dirty suds moving downstream? While it's okay with me to class that episode as merely a productive daydream, many say the dead are with us still and that concern for our welfare is the focal point of their afterlife.

But what if Wohler did something that *directly* set his descendant's behavioral decline in motion? Doesn't that then mean that he—a product of his times, to be sure—is responsible for what we've become?

Our one celebrity, he was supposed to be on our side.

Narcissus at home

"Dear old dad" (as he liked to refer to himself) was the real star of our show. The smarter than average bears of his day were fast being replaced by charming bears, such as movie stars, as the ones we held on high.

And so I remember the Clark Gable incident.

Heartthrob of the silver screen, his picture appeared in the newspaper again that day to the delight of one of my dad's bobby-soxed, hair-sprayed students. She cut out the photo, glued it to an index card, wrote "Mr. Elton, English Teacher," and placed it on his desk. My father couldn't wait to race home and share this delicacy.

He was a handsome guy.

Another student cloaked her feelings for him in an essay, a parody of some school-politics saga that cast the players as dog breeds instead of men. My father was the bulldog, "slim of hip," who saved the day. "Slim of hip! Slim of hip!" he crowed at home, while my mother fumed and I adored.

Elektra, they called me, sniggering—a funny batch of syllables, it didn't sound like a real girls' name. I guessed that whoever she was, Elektra had done something wrong.

"It's an old story," they said, "about a girl who loved her father a little too much." Was that the genesis of their practice that, as a toddler, I was taken to my father's bed every morning? My mother carried me in proudly, as though delivering expensive chocolates, and I was set sentry to watch my father awaken to the day.

In 1956 little girls throughout my neighborhood received similar lessons to worship daddy and discover their *feminine wiles*. Was it abuse? When I set out in earnest to find out what ailed us as a family, I looked to the head of household. Did he shape me as an Elektra, doomed to self-destruct? Did Sam and Ben de-potentate because they opted out of that sheer arrogance of entitlement?

After I was carried into his bed at dawn, and then called Elektra at breakfast, my parents would go on and on about how surely, as a teenager, I'd have so many boyfriends they'd have to *chain me to the radiator*.

One of my earliest memories is touring the house looking for the radiator. What I found, instead, were metal grates over holes on the floor where hot air entered. I pictured myself on a short tether of metal links, sitting there beside these furnace blasts while other people went to and fro. It was frightening. I felt guilty about my appearance, a topic my father focused on regularly; he ran to me in pride when a male friend of his commented favorably on my looks. I never believed it, because Sam and every other taunting boy in the neighborhood called us girls ugly punks every day. But were all fathers obsessed like this?

Narcissus needed a team in which no one broke ranks, along with a daily quota of compliments to meet the comfort zone. Like any parent, he expected his offspring to look up to him. How could one not love his warmth on the days when, quota filled to overflowing, he had something to give? How could an unformed soul, child in body and mind, avoid the pitfalls of self-hatred whenever he closed up again, leaking scorn, shutting the door, and retreating into literary thoughts?

Perils of early chemistry

Still. There had to be something, some event, some slip that set our bloodline's downward slide in motion. At work in his laboratory, might Wohler have inhaled or ingested something too fierce for his descendants' DNA? He and his kind were always blowing up things, breaking test tubes on themselves. Convalescing was part of the career. Could some toxin have penetrated his cells—something unseen, unstudied, that injured our genetic strand?

What if it came from dipping unprotected hands into the mercury trough, a common feature of laboratories in his day? The strange behavior of better-known chemists—Paracelsus, Isaac Newton—have been attributed to mercury poisoning.

The more I thought about my father, the more I lost my fervor to hang a dead man. Having discovered my own sensitivity to gluten and dairy products, my need for certain vitamins and minerals lest all hell break loose in my mind, I even toyed with striking the phrase "Wohler Madness" from my vocabulary. Allergies and nutrient deficiencies could be passed on genetically—and the environment was a teeming mess now, far more so than in Wohler's or even Agnes' day. Given these things, plus the incredible spike in "mental illness" worldwide, so poorly addressed by the broken dogma of psychiatry's "biochemical brain imbalance" theory, I had to question whether the special and tragic destiny I once called the family disease was really all that unique.

Perhaps, for us, Friedrich Wohler was simply the last productive stop on a larger, species-wide slip into narcissism, black depression, and schizophrenia. Like autism, these are disorders that throw a person's focus too perilously, and quite fearfully, on the self as separate from others. Parents of autistic children have a saying: We're all on the spectrum. Maybe we are all suffering from variations of biochemical impairment, thanks to the Industrial Revolution.

What would Wohler do?

One day, a thought came that shattered the protective layer of my daily life, fostering a mix of alarm and aha! It didn't jibe with the rancor I felt toward my father and pushed uncomfortably against that part of me that couldn't let him off the hook. It made a mockery of R.D. Laing and John Weir Perry's lauding of the visionary quality of madness (unless one could say that all illness has its vantage point from which we learn).

The idea, terrifying yet ripe with possibilities for global healing, also crowded out patriarchy as ultimate culprit. I began to seriously question whether male rule was first cause of a sick civilization, witch burnings, and mad women. The thought, as it took shape, went something like this: Could all "mental illness" and "behavior disorders" have an environmental root? Toxic planet, toxic mind?

If not for Nina, this connection would never have been made. I knew it was heresy, and all sorts of bad things happen to heretics.

Such a proposed link between mind/behavior and earth was blasphemous to conventional psychiatry with its burgeoning palette of new names for the same-old-drug approach to "brain disorders." It was also blasphemous to psychotherapists concerned about the drugging of our population, but convinced the talking cure was the only cure. It would surely be discounted by the remaining anti-psychiatry advocates, whose "mental illness" defines their oppression, their bid for civil liberties, their identity as individuals out of step with the status quo. And it deflated the romantic notion that madness can be a pretty groovy trip, with hidden gifts and silver linings.

Hey, I didn't ask to form this thought. I loved being a therapist, trancing to…wherever…and glimpsing the mythic components of a psychotic break. I didn't ask to end up with a child with autism, either. But her experience taught me to suspect a hidden truth about so-called mental illness. Toxic earth, toxic mind—and generations to come that will struggle with relationships, struggle to find their own equilibrium in so many ways, ways that will challenge the mind, the body, and all of our souls.

The facts of a personal life-change of such magnitude are hard to deny. I stopped having migraines, overcame the fear of many things and people, developed the capacity to sustain relationships, quit fantasizing, and finally stuck with a thought-train—all because I quit eating certain everyday foods, then proceeded to send nutrients and detoxifiers into my body daily. I was not the only one, I learned from the e-mail listserves. This should have been front-page news.

On the other hand, all it sounds so simple, the stuff of jokes. Must have been something you ate. The mighty mind will be disgraced if it's shown up by the gut, by hormones, by methylation byways. The scariest part is that not one professional helper, not one physician, told me to follow this path. Nina's experience showed me the way. The implications—that the mentally ill can heal themselves—fired my days with a troubling inner storm as I feared for a world that won't listen.

And yet, as I regarded the troubles among my family, I accepted at long last that I'm the one who lucked out.

If our special children really aren't a divine lesson, why won't science say what is scientifically so about them? Why the deluge of dollars for research into diseases that touch far fewer families? Why not come clean with what we've done to our children, and ourselves? And what about the rest of the lepers with labels? Why aren't schizophrenics, bipolars, ADHDers, and all the others up for the same overhaul in outlook?

Add one more subgroup, if researchers such as the Pfeiffer clinic are correct. Criminals are apparently the most toxic of the bunch. What does that make of the category we most love to hate?

What to make of the ancestor now? Wohler never knew it, but the field of organic chemistry that he helped set in motion was a direct hit to the behavior of our species.

Will the real scientist please stand up?

Chapter 18

NARCISSUS AND THE QUEST FOR INFAMY

There was a loose end that still needed resolving. Precisely how was I related to Friedrich Wohler? I wanted a familial tag by which to address him as I alternately vilified and admired him. But I was no good at genealogical search, so I hired an expert.

When I read the report, I felt a great shifting and breaking loose, like land masses dividing within me, an avalanche so unexpected I could only hang on for the ride.

No blood connection.

What? It was all a lie! Now I had to give up the favorite family dream, which assured us that although our bloodline might be jinxed, one among us could have the chance to be great. Some of us were and would be nuts; the family disease, we all figured, was just the way it was. If there were a counter-idea (a profound lack of nutrition affecting mind and behavior, a raging intolerance to some food that set the brain aflame, perhaps a thyroid malfunction or another non-judgmental, scientific explanation) we'd never been told. The presence of a founding father of Science in our past meant we needn't be bothered: we had him, the role model, the pinnacle that could be attained.

But no. It was only another dinner-table yarn told by my father to boost his inflated, precarious view of himself. The lie of Narcissus lived on, a special link that set us apart: madness, or genius?

Before this news, my father's pointless lies—his *exaggerations*—were minor blips on the radar of character. He boasted that his brother taught at Yale, when really it was a small private college in Connecticut. When I was pumping gas for a living in California, he assured cronies I was a "junior executive in an oil company." The size of our acreage grew and grew every time he described Kai's and my modest patch of land to his retired friends. There were more, but who can say if he even remembered them, even heard his lies as they left his lips? It was important to stay ahead of the pack, the average bears.

Who knows what he said about his *special* grandchildren. Mostly he avoided Nina, Pete, and Paul and lavished praise on Chucky, Ben's oldest (and neurotypical) son. The three *special* children were, well, deficient. He saved face by reminding others they were adopted: you paid your money, you took your chances.

Released

Who was I, if I wasn't separate from the average bears? Who was I if I wasn't connected to genius, awash in promise until the very end of a life that might never match Friedrich Wohler's output…*but could?* And what did the news make of my brothers, who also set themselves apart from others, save for the tribes each clung to: the "mentally ill" for Sam, the born-again Christians for Ben? Where each hunkered down in the safety of numbers, but secretly held themselves apart as not entirely one of the herd?

After a few embarrassed days of excommunication from the chemist's bloodline, I let myself take a full breath. First I attacked the clutter in my house, the piles I'd closed out of eyesight while pursuing my "special destiny." I wondered if I was trying to avoid a truth I could not process; cleaning and organizing brought control over the moment. I dived into the ordinary and took a certain shine to it. I was released from my obligation to redeem Wohler's legacy along with the concomitant wish for household servants so that I might draw up the grand design.

Cut loose from the family fantasy, easing back into the human race, at long last I could view people as a glorious collection of all kinds of bears. Each individual had a personal destiny that I could see now was not a subject for comparison. I had to become one in order to know that there really are no average bears, no flotsam and jetsam on which the intellectual elite rest their tender feet. That we all wander unwary into genius or madness, bad behavior or greatness, at those very individually cast intersections of body, mind, and spirit.

The relief endured. I was no longer torn in two over a choice between mundane obligations and miracles to perform. I wasn't wasting my time, not measuring up, under the gun. In fact, Time, a spare commodity while fighting autism, suddenly billowed, blossomed, and bubbled before me.

I wanted to thank the chemist's clan for letting me borrow him, but most of all for the lack of any tie at all.

Separating

In the end it wasn't the heart that stopped him, even after I'd tried so hard to shield it from my traitorous will and ideas. It was renal cell cancer.

There's a limbo when your dad's been dead for some time, but not recently dead or long-ago dead. People don't expect you to say much. You've bounced from the "grieving" category, but it's not over yet. It took me two years to reach finality. The other day, I almost missed him.

For weeks after the funeral I felt a great lifting up, as though I could do anything. Permission for full steam ahead, the long elusive jewel of Freedom placed in my bank vault at last. Soon, I realized I was *being* him—pushy, commanding, ideals first. Not exactly like being possessed by the dead, merely given the chance to try on their strong suit. But I had to admit that the point was to usurp, not to imitate. Itching to show him up, because that was never allowed. He was the last person I wanted to mimic.

How Robert Elton talked up his children to others, how marvelously we were conjured into air! His students and colleagues knew us as the apples of his eye. Many a comment, delivered in classrooms from which we were barred, floated back to ears that didn't know whether to turn red, or go in for a cleaning—had we heard that right?

I suspect this was harder on the boys than me. After all, I wanted to follow in his footsteps by teaching and writing. On the one hand, what greater flattery could there be—yet on the other hand, what if I surpassed him? Yet how could I? I was only a girl.

Our dad let us know that, although he didn't live up to family expectations of engineering endeavors or doctoring, he'd shown them all.

At least, he must have thought, *I will never contract the Wohler Madness.*

Such are the random pictures held by a daughter with a dad dead not very long, but long enough for the relationship to be, once and for all, over. You stop wondering if he's looking over your shoulder. You know what you have to do. Pull up the buried land mines and detonate them into neutral space. Complete a final review of how he praised or paralyzed you, then let it rest. Watch the way you watch the past, one last time. Finally I get to be his student, hoping that the long moratorium on these matters hasn't rendered the enigma impenetrable to analyze. It's so easy to pull apart the character of one who can no longer win the argument, a scoop of ashes among mausoleum shelves.

It's a coward's way out.

"My heart is torn by all I cannot save..."

This is how I will remember Sam: the man beneath the mental patient, striving for control of his care plan review. Indulged because he's crazy.

My brother has settled into nursing home life. Kansas is the only state to run Nursing Facilities for Mental Health (NFMH). Nuthouses, by any other name, moved into former geriatric facilities.

At first it was obvious Sam didn't need to be there. But his girlfriend did, and he wouldn't hear of leaving her side. I saw her flitting about the halls with ease, in clean clothes, while Sam was hunched over a walker, looking at the ground, his still-long fingernails dissected by lines of black dirt. *He's never going to stand erect again. He's never going to get out of there.*

Doctors decreed that Sam's pained gait was neurological in origin, and ever-higher doses of Neurontin were prescribed. Once I spoke to the NFMH's doctor about our father's bout with leg cramps, much like those that plagued Sam. "He went all over the country looking for an expert," I said to the silence on the phone line, "and finally a doctor at Yale put him on potassium and calcium." More silence. "Listen, if I don't take potassium before going to sleep I get charley-horses all night long. Our mom has terrible arthritis, too, as do I—but fish oil does the trick. I wonder if Sam could try it?"

"Oh, I take fish oil myself!" the doctor confided. "Because you never know." (About heart attacks, I assumed.) "Well, I suppose we could check his levels. But too much potassium is very dangerous," he warned.

I heard nothing more about it. Sam was in the dark about these possibilities when we convened for his review meeting. He had a page full of notes scribbled in his own hand.

We sat in an office located next to the main desk, in a former patient's room used for clerical overflow. The carpet was pink and filthy, the disarray months old. Since I attended many school meetings with Nina's "team," and there are so many team players, I expected a full room. But there was only one young nurse and a dietician in attendance for this review of Sam's past, present, and future.

The phone rang constantly with a piercing cry that irked Sam. Ditto when someone came in to collect folding chairs, banging the steel seats next to our ears. My brother nearly bit the guy's head off. This was his moment, one of few times when everyone agreed that it was all about Sam.

A few days ago I had read that Seroquel, Sam's main chemical straightjacket, was now one of the top litigated drugs in Pharma's arsenal. Patients on Seroquel, it turned out, experience nearly three and a half times as many cases of diabetes as those using older anti-psychotic drugs. The FDA was concerned enough to issue a MedWatch safety alert about the risk of hyperglycemia and diabetes for those taking it. The drug has also been linked to pancreatitis, a dangerous inflammation of the pancreas, ketoacidosis (a poisoning complication of diabetes), cardiac events, coma, and death. It starts sounding worse than Haldol, the drug that had carried Sam after Thorazine became passé. Sam became much more lucid and verbal without Haldol's "grinding noises" inside his head.

It hurt to sit in this dirty, disorganized room with the chubby young nurse, whose condescending Okie accent grated on my ears, and the silent dietician whom Sam complimented repeatedly about the food. It hurt, because they allowed him to feel important in his rambling when all three of us knew it was a story about nothing. It hurt because I was in on the game. Once more I betrayed my brother.

Sam convened our meeting because the nursing home had nothing to say. "You're stable, Sam," the nurse kept repeating, meaning *you don't give us any trouble.* What else can they muster up about such a nice guy, so thoroughly medicated that he never flips out?

Glancing at Sam's list, I was reminded of some other papers he had carried until they wore thin, number dances beyond my grasp. Sam on this day has the same blue-lined notebook paper, littered with hieroglyphs that mean something to him. But they are neither mathematical nor chemical shorthand.

Sam consulted his list of topics about Sam (health, disability, relationship with girlfriend), upon which no one offered comment. Sam had a lot to say, but it was like a UFO that refuses to land or fully show itself in the sky—you can't quite grasp what it *is.*

So I listen to his tone.

He could have been, as our father liked to say, *someone.* Sam the Brain sounded like a businessman, or an administrator, someone comfortable in the role of leader. He really did a good job, given that his material was nonexistent. That's when it struck me.

My brother, the eldest, was not a social misfit because he was a shy introvert. He was always primed to lead. He just couldn't make himself heard. He couldn't read people right, so when they wavered or disagreed, he assumed they hated him. Rather than kill them, he allowed the murder of his own soul.

This default position was modeled by Agnes and the other "mentally ill" in our bloodline. Those who are different are patently *wrong.*

I thought about Ben, hiding from life but looking good on the outside. As a boy, his one dream was to be an auto mechanic. It was a dirty, greasy job, ill respected, hardly good enough for our father. Ben took a degree in car dealership management and for years doled out foreign-car parts to customers whose pettiness and irritation drove him up a wall.

What might Sam have become? A spirited scientist? The writings on physics that seek to explain it to a hungry public sound more spiritual by the day. Where would my older brother be now, if his boyhood astonishment at the universe had been nurtured into a mystical mathematician?

And because each time I saw him I was shocked by how fast he had aged, how debilitated he'd become, I couldn't help but wonder: how will Sam die? A slow, excruciating death like our father, remaining suspicious of alternative medicine until it was too late to start?

What if the toxic load in Sam erupted into a similar plague? Would he lose his mind completely like our father in his final days, overwhelmed by pain and medications, seeing things that weren't there, trying for no reason to pull out his IV and run from the sickbed? Would Sam be attended, as was Narcissus to the end, by family and supportive hospice—or would we let the nursing home do the dirty work? Would I be able to avoid his last days, as I did in the case of our father, slowly drowning in fluid coming too fast for his body to clear? Perhaps I would only hear about it, yet never wipe from mind the image of his dead body lying on the mortician's slab, bright purple from suffocation.

Listening to my older brother trying to salve his dignity, clinging to superiority among his keepers, I realized that it was one thing to worry about the Earth, about humanity's probable fate, about whether the increasing toxic burden on the body robs us of the capacity for empathy. It was yet another thing to wonder, if Sam were well, whether he could escape becoming Narcissus Junior. In some ways, sitting there, I could see, beyond the toll taken by drugs, that he was the spitting image of our father.

Despite my great puzzlement that the nutrient path is not being shouted from the rooftops, I understood that full recovery takes more than detox and a diet that helps, rather than hinders, the gut-brain expressway. Once I came into the clearing and blinked at all the light, I still had to make major adjustments in my relationships, my language, and my use of the time newly freed up after so much "working on myself." I needed to learn remorse (not the same as paralyzing guilt) and reciprocity, and develop a slow, satisfying taste for redemption. I suspected that it would take more than nutrients for Sam to look out and see a world beyond his fantasies of greatness, and not be afraid. Old habits of relating to others die hard. Neither diet nor amino acids can effect, without conscious effort, a personality or soul overhaul. They only clear the way to greater responsibility for choices. They stop one from feeling *in overdrive but stalled,* or at least that was how it was for me.

But every time I saw Sam, a questioning voice would arise sooner or later. Why not me instead of him? Why was he there, at the behest of strangers? Why did he have only one small room with cement block walls? Why did the world have to lose one more physicist, one chemist who might have undone what the likes of Wohler set in motion? Sometimes I counted my mind as the lesser sacrifice, for Samuel was The Brain. What did I have to show, what had I done? Only slogged on, searching for love and truth and healing.

Sam the good boy (if rather shy), the brilliant Samuel, the last person in the world to touch a recreational drink or drug—was an addict whose soul had been sold to Pharma's profit machine and their assorted minions. In the end, Sam was a permanent resident in a place like this, one with dimly lit rooms, no classy glass lobby, no volleyball court on the grounds. Like Agnes, he submitted peaceably. He sat and smoked and doted on his girlfriend, his supreme tormentor and saving grace. My brother, the "mental health consumer," could still plead with the system for his fifteen minutes of dignity. At his care plan review meeting the staff and I colluded to keep it intact.

Can I tell him?

After he'd had enough, Sam thanked the attendees and struggled to regain his walker. As we crossed into the ward he said to me, "I think that was a good meeting."

We headed up the hall to the lobby. It was hard to find two empty seats where the television wasn't blaring. *What's the point of this mission?* I asked myself. I had only used the care plan review as an excuse to visit. What I really came for was to let Sam know that we are no relation to the chemist Friedrich Wohler.

What would the news about Wohler do for Sam? Where did I get off assuming that he would be as relieved as me? Would he throw his walker away, suddenly start making sense, and stride out of the place a new man?

Alternately, why did I worry it might slay him to find out that we were unrelated to genius, to sever the connection with a go-getter science guy he might have used to charge the batteries that at least got him through college? Why couldn't I simply imagine that he would be blasé about it all, chalk it up to family stories gone awry and forget about it?

I doubted that Sam would let me implicate our father and his need to lie in order to amplify our special-bear natures. I keep wondering why I was challenging his need for an untarnished monument to the man. Sam had so little—why barge in, bludgeon a memory, and leave?

Sam sat down gingerly as far as possible from the 5 o'clock news, with wheelchairs parked up close to the TV that no one was watching. I turned to face my brother, taking in the emaciated, nearly toothless features.

"Hey," I touched his arm. "I came here to tell you something."

Samuel Elton peered up at me from his bent penance and did his best to look me in the eye. In the space of that glance, I learned one thing: Sam, Nina, my Cambodian-American nephews—and yes, even the spirit of my father, Robert Elton—are my tribe.

A long pause before I could get the words out.

"Mur's driving up in two weeks. We'll come to see you. We'll go out for dinner."

✳ ✳ ✳

As late fall leaf-coloring began in the heartland, the nursing home notified us that Sam was speaking incoherently, urinating on himself, and combative with the staff. Their response was to send him to a bona fide mental hospital. Before Christmas he would be admitted three more times. "Four hospitalizations I really didn't understand" was the closest he'd ever get to criticizing his keepers.

After he was "stable" again, I took my brother and his girlfriend out to eat. Sam's right arm hung limp in his lap. "Can't use it. All part of the legs and back problem," he stated, wolfing down a cheeseburger. He was more hunched over than ever, his back at a nearly 45 degree angle. In the car where we waited—and waited—for his girlfriend to shop Wal-Mart, Sam drooped uncontrollably against Nina, unable to stay upright. She poked at him, giggling, calling him "Funcle Sam!" But Sam was fast asleep. Saliva poured from his mouth just as it had when he was awake—if that's what you could call his ever more slurred and slouching state.

Pulling Nina into the front seat with me, I closed my eyes and asked, "My Goddess, my All, what can I do?"

I had just put forth a tentative suggestion about some nutrients that might help his legs and back. It was now many years after the Pfeiffer trip, and this time I proposed to lobby his regular MD. Dr. Botchkin, Sam's immovable psychiatrist, was many miles from the nursing home and less involved in his protocol now.

"I've already talked to your doctor—he said he takes fish oil himself!" I told Sam.

"Write it all down and I'll go over it with him," Sam said. At which I waffled.

Write a list, pretty much Greek to my brother, which he would either lose or present without the proper mix of conviction and tact? Not that I believed we had much of a shot. But how could I trust Sam? Was he still capable of making sound decisions?

So I said I'd work on it. Before leaving the restaurant, I also proposed to take him to a reputable chiropractor whose patients included university athletes and other healers from my area. Days later, true to form, Sam denied both offers.

Everyone's choices are complicated. Sam did as his girlfriend commanded, and she had clearly hated the Pfeiffer vitamins, calling them "a disaster." Who in Sam's position would turn down the so-called "love" she offered him? The love of his life kept her balance by continually jockeying for control, and a truly and fully recovered Samuel could end that for her. Yet how could I come between him and the only person he'd ever deeply connected with for the long haul?

But could I stand by and watch my brother slowly die of unaddressed *physiological* crises mislabeled as *mental* illness? I had considered a legal arrangement assigning me as guardian-conservator, but that option weighed hard. How could I take my brother's freedom away and disrupt his romance unless I were sure I could make good on the benefits of the non-drug path?

In every crisis that twists my gut and mars the heart with helplessness, I turn to this verse as a last resort for letting go. I penned it the day after I could not convince an "alternative" newspaper to cover the story of our Pfeiffer involvement and how the system let Sam down.

PRINCIPLES OF NONATTACHMENT

What to do when someone you love
would rather be sick than make a stand?
Hold to your truth at bone-level—
in the face of their stone walls, the harm
done by a hand you cannot stay,
the wide-eyed stare that scarcely masks
just how insane they think you are.
Give to yourself the gift of listening.
Stop trying to fix your family,
for if they can't share
the habit of trust with you,
they know only that there is
one black sheep in every bunch.
Forget them with compassion.
Move on with heart tuned for the one
voice you can hear with all the pride
of your mad perseverance—
no tricksters,
no trance,
no flaming angels.
It's you.
When family doesn't listen,
it only matters that you do.

PART FIVE
FOR LOVE OF THE LIFE FORCE

Chapter 19
MADWOMEN THEN AND NOW

It was time to run another ad for a respite worker to assist us with Nina's care. I was notorious for hiring the first person that called. Each time I swore I wouldn't act desperate, but this time the applicant sounded so good. When she showed up—a gal my age that lived close by, claiming prior experience with autism—I hired her on the spot.

We seemed to have so much in common. She said she completed her history degree by writing a major research project on the Salem witch trials. She wanted to start a women's group in the county. She was an artist who drew mothers as trees. I was vexed when Nina didn't warm up to her, for I was giddy with the prospect of having a new friend who got paid for coming over.

But Nina is able to read a person's core. This time, I overlooked my daughter's cold shoulder toward the stranger. Our family would pay, dearly.

It didn't take long before Diana's stories began to shift. Before I knew it, her degree was in art, not history. She had worked for the CIA, then it was the LAPD. Her parents were the picture of healthy, nutritious eating and living, yet they were hateful, rigid, and insane. She got premonitions about when people were going to die.

It didn't take long before the woman was forthcoming about all the psychiatric medications she swallowed to make it through each day. She alluded to wearing diagnoses of schizophrenia, then bipolar. But by then I was an enabler.

I spent hours bolstering Diana's self-esteem with pep talks, loaning her books, taking her to movies and women's groups. Her husband was disabled and could barely work; they lived on the poverty line. Kai and I gave them food; later, I found she'd helped herself to batteries and light bulbs too. After all, she was always being "screwed" by someone: her landlord, her husband's boss, the Social Security Administration.

I tried often to talk to her about nutrients—what they'd done for me, what they did for Nina. She stuck to her story about her crazy, unloving parents running a health food store (albeit in a tiny, backwoods town); because of their "enforced" natural remedies, she preferred not to go the nutrient route. The constant presence of her sad, little-girl demeanor was a powerful picture. Diana believed she had lost her chance at life.

Hindsight is horrible. On some level, she was Sam. I was going to get her through this, though I could not save my brother. But Sam would have never done what she did.

All expenses paid and more

Nina was in pain. Shortly after each meal, she rolled into a ball or screamed and kicked. She had to stand to move her bowels. They were extremely slow to get in motion. All the gains we'd made with chelation were not so much lost as superseded. A new clinic promised treatment for autistic children with severe gut problems. We decided to travel to Texas and have Nina's gut scoped by a gastroenterologist who understood autism.

Kai couldn't get away, and Diana seemed the perfect choice to accompany me. I knew she was dying to take a vacation. When I asked her to come to Texas, her eyes lit up as if contemplating a cruise. All expenses paid.

After I steered the rental car out of the Austin airport, it was time to find grub. What with Nina's and my diet, restaurant choosing was a careful art. We picked Indian food, to Diana's delight. The place was a little more upscale than I'd planned, but Nina behaved and what the heck, it *was* a vacation of sorts. That point of view continued through many other restaurants, more than I could really afford, during our stay.

The next morning we drove to a health food store to purchase the broth and hard candy that Nina would be allowed during the "clean out" before surgery. It was then that I realized my mistake. In the car, on unfamiliar streets when I sorely needed navigational help, Diana fell apart.

"I have nothing! My teenagers are lazy as sin. They're drama queens who remind me of me! Our landlord is so out to get us! And it's always been like this," she wailed, tears flowing down red cheeks, her already little-girl look more pitiful than ever.

Still in savior mode, I tried to bolster a bright side, listing her pluses, her potential to endure. Diana, however, freed from the overflowing chaos of her everyday life, was no longer distracted from the void within; it rushed in to fill up the space in her mind, front and center.

The time came to go inside the store, where I needed her help with Nina while scouting the aisles. Diana blew her nose elaborately, her face a resentful mask. She closed the discussion with, "At least you have a house and a car!"

She stayed up all night in the hotel lobby, while Nina crowded me to the edge of our king size bed.

The next morning, before our initial foray to the clinic, Diana was all smiles. She informed me she was going to sit in a nearby cemetery and sketch. Whoa! There was no time clock, but I'd counted on a mutual understanding of our tag-team responsibilities. I again needed a navigator to help me find my way across this foreign city and locate the clinic for the first time. It would be a challenge to do that and handle Nina, too. Diana groused and took the map, which she had no knack for reading.

I'd pictured her sharing more than just the vacation aspect of this trip with me. I had assumed she'd share every trial with me, including while Nina was in surgery. Nina was terrified and it infected me. I could have used some understanding, or at least dependability and presence. Instead, I silently asked myself why I'd brought Diana along.

My respite worker spent the rest of the day walking through museums and the capitol building, savoring the flair of Austin, Texas. During the entire trip, I was relieved of Nina-duty for only about two hours. I didn't dare ask Diana to go with me the day of the surgery. She was fresh out of compassion for my fear about the procedure and Nina's plight, as she ping-ponged between agony over her own life and cavorting like a kid playing hooky. I suffered alone at the clinic when Nina was wheeled away, screaming, on a gurney, and when she fought and wept in the recovery room, frightened by IV needles in her arm. I cried to Kai over the phone when the diagnosis of autistic enterocolitis, well on her way to Crohn's disease was leveled at last, with no "friend" at my side to comfort me.

I knew then that she had to go. Out of our home, for good. I didn't need one more person to take care of, someone who in my loneliness I had fancied as a friend, but who couldn't do "friend." Kai was also putting on the pressure to ditch her, even while chatting amiably to her face. Was it her medication that blocked her from gaining insight into her own repetitive, chaotic ways? She seemed devoid of the Sam affect—there was no slur, no slowness of thought trains. Yet while she could *act* concerned for brief and convincing periods of time, real empathy was lacking. Nina continued to treat her like a piece of furniture. I continued to enable her.

The unease that built up for months could be summed up by a single phrase I often shared with Kai. Thanks to Diana, the madwoman so frequently in our home, our entire family had been taken hostage. We had to listen to her rage about a shifting crew of persons and authority figures she felt had mistreated her. But with the winter holidays ahead I couldn't afford to lose help with Nina, in whatever form.

✳ ✳ ✳

Christmas approached, the one holiday Nina enjoyed with all her might. Diana made sure we knew her family couldn't buy a tree, let alone afford gifts. She became increasingly surly about the holidays. It's a hard time for many (and adopting a Scrooge attitude is hardly rare), but I tried nevertheless to stay low-key about our preparations and plans.

I kept mulling over whether letting her go was imperative, telling myself there were still some positives. For example, Diana made us dinner, cleaned up the dishes, and did laundry at every turn. In fact it seemed she would rather do housework than spend quality time with Nina. "Well," I told myself, "it's so hard to get good people all the way out here in the country. Besides, Nina is crabby because of her gut pain." She even cleaned up Nina's copious diarrhea without complaint, even though some days she had to race home and take a shower. I was still, when I wanted to be, very good at tuning out what I didn't want to see. I did it because of the rapes.

Diana said there had been two. I never felt this story was a fabrication, for it didn't shift and eddy like the others; her pain was real. I assumed that being a rape victim at a tender age could addle a mind and heart irreparably. I continued to calm Kai down when he complained about her constant lateness, car troubles, and family uproar. To me, somehow, she was a sister who was oppressed and I owed her allegiance. The way that Narcissus sexualized Elektra held no candle to what she went through.

It was as though I shelved all I'd learned about giving up madness. I fell back on my rusty therapist techniques, but she sidestepped them—maybe I simply wasn't good enough to reach her. I could see the damage done to her by patriarchy. I accepted that the secret Freud covered up best—that of widespread sexual molestation of girl children—was the root of her malaise.

Inquisitors at the door

After yet another episode involving lies, tardiness, and stolen money, Diana and I closed the door to the den and sat down. She wept but agreed we should part ways. "Let's just get through the holidays," I suggested, making no move to downplay my need for assistance during this stressful time. She agreed that the timetable made sense.

The next day, I got a call from Nina's case manager.

"What's going on out there? I heard from Diana. Sue, she's going to turn you guys in!"

"Turn us in? For what?"

"To Child Protective Services, for child abuse! She cites 'philosophical differences' between the way you handle Nina, and what she thinks should be done. I don't know if she's bluffing or what."

"Well you've met her," I managed to say, frozen to my spot on the couch. "You know she's got big problems. You even mediated one of our disagreements. You know she's on some pretty stiff medication. Who's going to believe her?"

The social worker had known us for years. "Of course she's got problems. I'm not even supposed to be telling you about this. But I wanted to alert you."

"What do I do?"

"Hope it's just a case of her needing to talk to me. Maybe that was enough."

The same afternoon Diana showed up for work with a fine poker face. Nina and I were gone. Kai confronted her, without implicating the case manager, but the madwoman was anything but dumb. She blew. After raging at Kai for a full five minutes she slammed out the door, turning back to shake both fists at the house. "I'll get you!" she yelled.

The next day I picked up the phone after caller ID showed me Diana's number.

"My husband and I were running some figures, and I never got paid for my hours in Austin," she said.

To this day, I wonder if there could have been any other way to defuse her besides paying cash. It was preposterous, extortion at best, but I was adamant. She would not bilk us for a trip for which she was paid handsomely, and for which she gave little real work in return. "Diana, you were paid in salary and in so many other ways. Don't forget all the nice restaurants, your explorations of Austin—" Click! She hung up on me.

If we'd doled out even more dollars to avoid being "turned in," would it ever have been enough? We had to break the hostage mold.

Christmas was five days away, with Kai sharing time caring for Nina. I was glad it was just us. In light of the threat, we needed to pull in as a family. It had been two days and no word yet from investigators of child abuse.

The morning of the winter solstice everything changed. The Inquisitors came to the door.

Kai was headed out of town but I reached his cell phone just before his plane took off. *What do I do?*

"Cooperate," he said. He made the flight wondering if he'd return home to a house without Nina.

I put down the phone, sure I'd never get through this without him.

Luckily a new caregiver was in our home that day, and she had helped me clean up Nina's messes. Out of school already for winter break, Nina played on her bed in a cheerful, calm mood. When I saw the beat-up old car in the driveway I cursed, thinking it was one of Kai's clients showing up unannounced. So I asked Judy, the new gal, if she could find out what they wanted.

"We just want to see if Nina is okay." The Child Protective worker stood beside the special investigator, an unemployed cop the State had hired to help with the burgeoning number of these types of complaints.

"There's nothing wrong with her," said Judy defensively, barring the door and telling them to wait. She fetched me with a worried look.

The holiday horror show

"Oh, I know why you're here," I said, trying to be light-hearted. "Yes, we have a disgruntled former employee. She threatened to do this. Come on in." The two of them were blank. Later, I found out they were sent without any knowledge of the allegations. Always made anonymously, of course.

I still can't recall every detail about that hour during which I was ordered away from my child and questioned by the special investigator, actually a pretty nice guy from California. He set me at ease immediately, so I told him everything. He seemed especially keen to hear all about the clinic in Texas. I told him Diana accompanied us, I mentioned extortion—but he wanted the names of all Nina's doctors. He said he would contact her school as well; I was mortified. He asked me how she was disciplined. He was easy to see through when he was probing for something amiss. In the end he thanked me for the opportunity to learn so much about autism.

I wondered what was going on in Nina's room. I told him about the bite marks the social worker would find on our daughter's arms, self-injurious behavior caused by gastrointestinal distress. "She's way ahead of you," he assured me, referring to his colleague in the other room. "She knows how to spot that."

I could hear Judy in the kitchen banging pots and pans, making Nina's lunch loudly as a form of nonverbal protest. I was glad one of us could telegraph our real feelings.

In due time they left. Without Nina in tow, thank Goddess. While they wouldn't come right out and say *we found nothing*, I thought the worst was over. But the final decision was postponed by the winter break.

As we opened gifts from Santa, there was the specter of the almighty State removing Nina from our lives. Would her nutrient protocols be followed in foster care? Kai and I argued over everything during the thirty days it took for the system to make up its mind. Other faceless players within the State needed their turn at the seemingly endless stream of paperwork—after they had enjoyed their nice Christmas vacation, of course. Finally, we received written notice: **Unsubstantiated**.

The special investigator came out toward the tail end of this saga to "talk to the father." He apologized to Kai for the whole ordeal and said he would enter Diana's name into the system, flagged as a false reporter. We found the charges that she leveled more perplexing than anything Diana had done: *medical and emotional abuse*.

Nina's caseworker, free now to speak fully, elaborated on her initial contact with Diana about turning us in. "She believes you should spank Nina. Restrain her. She says it's emotionally abusive not to set limits with force. She definitely believes you should have put her on drugs."

"What, even after going to Austin with us? She knew what lengths we went to get Nina well. *Medical* abuse? This is too bizarre."

"She mentioned Prozac. Risperdal. To calm her down. She says Nina should get prescriptions."

The veil between my Habitat past and Nina's now seemed to be growing thin. Drugs to the rescue—not for the sake of the drugged, but for the benefit of their aides. Déjà vu. Thankfully we were exonerated. Had something gone amiss, had Nina been taken from us, I knew what would happen. Children in foster care are the most drugged in America. I couldn't let myself imagine her in chemical straightjackets just so the new people around her could cope. I knew she'd fight, but toxins level the soul and spirit while taking the body down, one side effect after another. Nutrients repair, but there's no profit in that. Diana was savvy enough to know that natural treatments were still viewed as a crackpot endeavor at large, upping her chances of snaring us for our "health food" ways.

Over time I came to hope that Diana's bold move made up for the rapes, that sense of powerlessness she had endured—a mix of genuine hard luck and the habit of drawing it to oneself. She was but one of many unloved, incested, abused, and depressed women who needed healing. One day, I believed, she would be ready to embrace it.

I also hoped for another silver lining: that I'd finally learned my lesson. *Don't try to save Sam by proxy.* How could I hate the woman? I *did* have something rich that she did not possess. I was gaining in understanding about just how pervasive and complicated the roots of madness can be.

※ ※ ※

A different time. Different complaints, different restraints. But then, as now, women made up the majority of the labeled mad.

As a young girl, my grandmother Agnes Wohler pieced together her days at the piano. Her parents procured lessons—not an easy task in rural Kansas, but a neighbor taught and loaned instruction books. Agnes wove fragments and techniques, popular songs and sonatas, into a full repertoire. Her parents said *practice every day.* Their daughter lost herself in the music without a glance at the clock.

Usually, when she practiced, she could hear her mother. Scraping at a corroded pan. Scratching a broom over parquet. Cleaning shelves, moving boxes. The faint background was complement, not competition. That's why Agnes stopped short one afternoon when silence intruded.

She knew she'd been keeping track of her mother for some time now, only to relax at the keys. Where she could hear a mother being just that, attacking disorder instead of staring, pained, at nothing. But one afternoon, in between the arias that Agnes loved that week, the absence of mother sounds assailed her. She flew off the bench.

Through every room, where sisters and a brother played or made themselves scarce, she hunted. Father was at the pharmacy, doing his work. In the kitchen, where Mother presided, Agnes found no trace. Except for the cellar door, ajar, and that was wrong.

Agnes descended, calling out as she dipped into dimmer light. No answer. The open door handed down a little daylight, but Agnes was drawn to where the quiet lay deepest. There by the washtub she saw her mother, her face frozen on a scream. For the woman had managed to drink the greater portion of a gallon of lye.

I imagine it was all she had at hand, in that moment when she finally ascertained that to climb those stairs once more was far worse than befriending her own death.

In the obituary she is named only "Mrs. Wohler."

The obit also says that Agnes didn't make it to the funeral (nor did two other sisters), due to "illness." Was this the beginning? Was this the trigger that sent Agnes slipping towards depression and self-hatred?

Did she wait until she was roughly the same age as her mother, hemmed in by parenting and sorrow, feeling like Jezebel and holding onto the thought of suicide like an addiction, a salve, a way out of this hate, hate, hate for the self. Later Agnes' man (who married sister Antonia first and then, when she died, offered the honor to Agnes) would coin the term: *the Wohler Madness*. All the children of the lye-drinker and her pharmacist husband ("druggist," in the day's vernacular) had it, even the one male who—while a practicing dentist—shot himself in the head.

So the *Wohler Madness* it was. Named by the outsider, the savvy Elton newcomer who pulled two of the female brood out of the house and into his bed. He could not, however, engineer a solution to their unremitting sensitivity, their pain, their need to be needed. The bloodline was still poison.

Her name was Bertha

For years, this was the story I told myself about Agnes: loss, grief, a heart punctuated by sorrow again and again, until the mind unhinged. Her mother, her sister, her beloved. It drove her mad. But spreading from that root was another patch of ground from which to dig for the truth about madness. *Oppression* was a word I learned from the B-Brothers concerning the Vietnamese, the poor and minorities. When I applied it to the female at large, and in particular to the women they knew, my revolutionary mentors squirmed.

I recall two things about the first women's liberation meeting I attended. One was the tenor of my fear on the walk over to the college campus. I'd been reading the works of the sisterhood for so long that the key authors seemed like friends. I'd battered Chris Glen with feminist rhetoric until he could recite it backwards. In public he appeared supportive: "I'm a lesbian trapped in a man's body," he'd say in the right quarters with all seriousness, fishing for what he could catch. Anger at his duplicity and the realities of oppression should have made me fly with righteous satisfaction toward the meeting room that day.

But if my legs were weak and my feet felt disconnected, my thoughts were a veritable study in repression-meets-oppression. I wouldn't let it surface, but the 1950's good girl in a navy Catholic school uniform kept trying to bump me off the sidewalk. Was I afraid of what I'd find when the meeting commenced—or of who I'd be forced to become, once it was over?

Chris raised no opposition to me going. I slammed out in my usual huff but soon took to dawdling, watching a squirrel dart, listening to a jukebox sounding faintly from within a neighborhood bar. As my stomach flipped and flopped I asked myself, *Are you a feminist or not? Or*—to use my father's worst epithet—*a phony?*

Inside the meeting room at last, there was no balm. The faces were grim. These women were college students, barely older than me, but it seemed as if they had lived so much more. No one smiled. *How refreshing,* thought Rebel Girl, *women don't need to smile and make nice just to set others at ease, just to show we're one-down!* But Catholic Girl worried: *This means they don't like me.*

The meeting began with talk that was no-nonsense and brave. I had overwhelming urges to smile, but instead I studied the participants for clues as to how to maintain the proper arrangement of my face.

The agenda has been lost to time, but it was action-oriented. This was no sharing of feelings in a consciousness-raising group; it was about gaining rights, either for ourselves or on behalf of oppressed women in our community. When it was over, I had done it. I had not smiled, I was initiated, I would never be the same. After the meeting I gave back to Chris all his socialist and Black Panther books. There! Now I was enrolled in the *real* vanguard!

Will Nina ever understand a word of this tale? Neither Agnes Wohler nor Marie Elton had one like it to offer me. They defaulted to *stand by your man*. But my great-grandmother's suicide, verified by the weekly obituary, held the key. To her community she was only "Mrs. Wohler," the one who married in. But her name was Bertha.

Madness descends mostly upon the loser in the gender wars. Statistically, women far outnumber men in their seeking of psychiatric help.

In 1972, a psychologist named Phyllis Chesler detailed what I considered to be the final word (at that time) on the Wohler Madness. Her premise was that, instead of genuine maternal nurturing, mothers often taught their daughters to play the subservient female role marked by constraint and self-sacrifice. The daughters often reacted later on in life as either "depressed" (their punishment if they were failures at this role) or "schizophrenic" if they outright rebelled in a most *un-ladylike* way.

This cast a sudden new light on my 1969 diagnosis. Perhaps it wasn't just a handy hereditary tag based on what my parents told the Habitat staff about the Wohler Madness. I didn't yet know anything about feminism, but I was mouthy and headstrong.

Chesler connects the dots in her own words:

> Women who reject or are ambivalent about the female role frighten both themselves and society so much so that their ostracism and self-destructiveness probably begin very early. Such women are also assured of a psychiatric label and, if they are hospitalized, it is for less "female" behaviors, such as "schizophrenia" and "promiscuity."

Bertha, however, had a pack of children to deal with. What rebellion was possible for an overtaxed housewife in a lonely Kansas town, circa 1918? Nothing but going gruesome into that good night, and so Bertha, no matter how she might have acted out previously, chose depression as her final will and testament. How could Agnes ever qualify for "nurtured" with an absence like that in the middle of her girlhood? She was marked—but not by bad mothering, I told my-self after Chesler's work became my new bible. She was dismantled by the hand of patriarchy clenching tighter and tighter around her life.

This feminist analysis of the roots of madness was one more cher-ished pearl that my experiences with Nina expanded into something greater than simply Mars versus Venus. William Walsh, that Pfeiffer researcher who discovered the copper overload danger in autistics, found the same problem in post-partum women. According to Walsh, post-partum depression is caused by an excess of copper that needs to be chelated by zinc—perhaps not the same heavy dosage, but one similar to children on the autism spectrum.

What if this was Bertha's final undoing—eight children in and out the womb? Or could it have been her husband's inadvertent fault as the local pharmacist? As glib to the dangers as Wohler the Old World chemist, did he inadvertently expose his wife and children to some slow poison thought to be as harmless as milk?

Or was it a combined assault, I asked myself, still not wanting to reduce everything to biology. Did Bertha represent a mind caged by the female role, a body susceptible to fatigue and stress, and a spirit crushed by Lutheran allegations of sin?

Bertha and Agnes. You don't hear those names for girls anymore. But I won't forget them.

Chapter 20
MOON RELATIONS

I've looked at madness from most sides now. Ditto many changes of heart on the topic of mothers, particularly my own.

Though she did it without pills, shock treatments, or extended hospital stays, it was Marie Elton, once Agnes the Wohler-mad left us, who took up the full brunt of the martyr's cross. I adopted what seemed to be the prevailing attitude in the family towards her: light to heavy contempt, studded with stretches of sheer neglect of her presence. I needed to be smarter than the average bear, and she forever told us that she was not. She was emotional; she cried with ease. As the only girl-child, I risked losing my sliver of self-respect if I didn't separate from the open hurt at the way her family treated her, and from her total letting down of the guard to reveal pain that was neither cardiovascular like her man's, nor scary like the addled Agnes. It was feminine, telegraphed the men in the family, who modeled to me the appropriate disrespect for her mere mother-being.

And yet, I was her sole heir to femaleness. Her daydreams centered on raising the happiest family ever, eternally close every minute of the day. Yet love, her ultimate goal, seemed to elude her. My fervent wish was not to settle for the same fate, and speeding through a stack of lunkhead boyfriends gave me the illusion of being proactive.

Then, during my years in the People's Republic of San Francisco, feminism provided a "click." My mother was oppressed! It was my task to educate her. Alas, she never followed me into the streets in protest, never joined a NOW chapter or read the books that prompted massive "clicks" in woman after woman around the globe. The whole thing made her nervous, and she much preferred novels to nonfiction. Her lack of strength and decisiveness fed my perennial scorn, which covered up the real loss: we never stood together on the same side of a single issue.

Phyllis Chesler had one thing right. The lack of strong guidance from the first female mentor could leave a gal ever so depressed, or so rebellious against the maternal example, that folks called the daughter insane.

So what came next, a widening of view, was a welcome change of heart. The Goddess awakening brought honor to mothers. It challenged me to see the womb as more than a bloody hovel to claw one's way through, delivered from primal ooze into the light. I became truly humbled by how my mother's womb gave me life, and understood her many years of trying to embody maternal prowess for the neighbors, for herself. After my miscarriages, pregnancy zoomed to an even higher pedestal. I reflected that my own mother knew mysteries I would never fathom.

Until my father's death, the bulk of thoughtful interaction between my mother and I centered on Narcissus (she in his unwavering defense, me the wronged party, out for reparations). In the long run, I still explain her shortcomings via the man she married. While my father lived, he mediated her responses. Her ease with disempowerment remains so thorough, so convincing, that even today one almost forgets she's a widow, a free agent grappling with responsibility to self and others.

Was she ever aware of her responsibility for Sam? Once, I asked her why she let him wear those shabby, peer-repellant clothes as a teen. Why didn't she notice he had no friends? "We thought he would grow out of it." *We.* Narcissus still lived.

I've always been taken care of, she's taken to saying and adds, with a heavy heart, *and I regret it.*

Good grief, she's 82 years old! Her formative years were spent being seen and not heard. Next, a stint as decorative object and breeder, a long-term career as a mother, then a reprieve when she obtained her degree and found a teaching job, followed by retirement as the Invisible: an elder female.

My mother is a widow managing money for the first time ever, terrified of its ebb and flow. But it doesn't take cash to be a mother-warrior, a parent-advocate facing psychiatrists and nursing-home administrators. Hence, when Marie Elton declines to step up for Sam, the excusers that constitute her family and friends wonder why I bristle. Occasionally she calls Sam's case manager, leaning on him as once she relied on the judgment of her husband. Why does my mother only obey men in authority, like a good girl?

Does it all spiral back to the watchful eyes of an exacting Father God? When I was Nina's age, kneeling day after day in my Catholic school pew, I knew the point was being good to buy favor, or relative safety. Because once a month—and how I dreaded it—the sisters would haul us to the sanctuary after lunch to make our confessions. I worried because I'd forget my sins and how many times each one. So I made them all up, apparently thereby sinning again. This proved I was defective, but I could always try harder to try to please next month. Except that I forgot to tally and keep track. Once freed from the confessional, I didn't want to think about those dark curtains with the unseen, priestly voice loud enough behind screen and scroll.

When I started to suspect that church might be more than a peripheral crutch for the weak, that it might really be a persuasive vehicle for the strong, I looked at such buildings with more fear than I ever knew during prepubescent mass. How little I wanted to go inside those massive doors ever again. Simply walking by a church I got the heebie jeebies. The intellectual and spiritual descendants of the Inquisition ran the place!

By then, however, I'd been moon-read by a divine maternal power, literally in my own grassy yard. As a result, I became convinced not only that spirituality was *the* cure for Crazy, but that women were better people. *It's patriarchy*, I believed with fervor, *that makes humanity one big dysfunctional family. Men are to blame. Inferior beings. Violent. Out of control.*

And yet: if our mothers sided with the worst of what patriarchy had to offer, they may still deserve a special permit. Not quite guilty, perhaps, but not innocent either.

Why is it we can't get past the failings of our all-too-human mothers? Why the enduring fury, ambivalence, guilt, and other emotions which refuse to heal? Without knowledge of our true Female history, Her story that was once cherished by both women and men, perhaps we want too much from one woman after that mystical act whereby we traveled the length of her womb. Because we can't recall what it was like to have the Divine Mother as a simple fact of earthly and spiritual life, we can't let our mothers off the hook for not measuring up.

The minister who counseled the mother of my old Pagan mentor Cedar Wing had it backwards. We don't conjure up the Divine Feminine because mothers fail—instead, we besiege our mothers for divine perfection because we can't recall what it was like when God was female, and ever so present in the myth-loving mind.

Gender bender

But then with Nina came a crash course in the power of a toxic planet to derail the love of learning and the basics of friends and family. Thrown against the wall of my supposed superiority, a cascade of outdated thoughts crumbled down. Stepping out of the rubble, I learned that men aren't messed-up, hormonal mistakes of nature that we can merely hope to mollify if we're to live with them. As the epidemic of violence and behavior disorders spreads like brush fire to even the richest homes, it becomes clear that men are the more vulnerable beings.

Suffering autism-spectrum disorders four times as often as girls (not to mention their greater numbers pinned to a flurry of acronyms like ADD, ADHD, OCD, ODD, PDD, ED and CD), our boys are explained away by (male) social scientists sexing the brain. *We can't help it! We have heaps of testosterone directing our big hairy selves!* Meanwhile, endocrinologists use male rats and male puppies to troubleshoot how chemicals effect reproductive problems. Lowered sperm count is now a fact for humanity worldwide. Birth statistics confirm it: we are slowly turning the planet female. A disruption of the fetal hormone system by chemicals shows a striking new gap in the male-female birth ratio. With one gender's greater susceptibility in our toxic age, how could the male mind not snap? If men are more vulnerable, in many ways, to the substances that humans are cavalier about messing with—and which affect their behavior—then surely they need much more than a *(wink, wink)* "boys will be boys."

It may be that the two sexes are not really alien to one another, Venus and Mars trying to make the best of it. The only way we differ may lie in our ability to detox, at least as children. This is but one of many mindbenders that forces me to rethink the men of my bloodline.

The fractured I-Thou of a people poisoned

Some say autism is more pronounced, symptom-wise, in girls. If males are extra-susceptible to the contaminants of a post-modern society, how much body-burden did it take to fling Nina past the natural protection of estrogen into the full-scale attack of an autoimmune response? Is this why I can't bring her, fully, back to us?

Yet Nina, a child assailed by toxic metals, stealth viruses, whacky bacteria, and who-knows-what synthetic industrial stew, makes it possible for me to think about my brothers in a new way. Nina either fails to notice a social shun or, when she gets it, wears a puzzled face so forthrightly that an observer's heart breaks. She takes me back, way back, to my brothers as young and vulnerable boys, not yet schooled in the ways of shutting out and shutting down. She sends me to a land of terrifying remorse over the great arcing waves of distance that lay between us when they needed me most.

I dug through many theories looking for the roots of the Wohler Madness, only to end up questioning if my brothers and I were ever truly in the running for *mental* illness at all. Given what Nina has taught me about my own mind-body issues, I now ask whether Sam, Ben, and I could have been toxic kids.

True to family form, none of us ever mention the Wohler Madness. Since our father's death we not yet shared one word about him, the lucky one who was spared. Or was he? Narcissus by choice? Or something else?

The standoff with my brothers endures, with our infrequent phone calls, holidays apart, and unshared lives bricking up the walls that only adults within a family can maintain.

Listening to autism

They are the distant men I cannot free.

Nina is the light I will let no label extinguish.

My daughter is the spirit of wildlife caught in human form, as all children are. Yet Nina has not learned the self-conscious ways of society. She walks naked onto the front porch. She poops on the floor. She sings to console herself because she has discovered it works. She strokes water because it flickers, supple and easy to befriend. She rubs her vulva on Orange Kitty in full view because I can't convince her that people don't want to see that.

But she *does* care a fig for what you think—if she knows you, if you mean something to her. Lately I see her studying my face. She is trying to grasp my humanity; I feel it. It's more than looking to see if I'll give her the cookie or not. Something is afoot. It always is. Nina can be envisioned as developmentally delayed, behind. Or she can be seen for the phenomenon that she is: change, growth. It's part of her message: *We are "afflicted," but we too strive to thrive.*

And Nina, just in case you ever read this (still a strong possibility, considering I once figured you'd never speak, and considering how much you adore books), I want you to know how much I love it when we laugh. At the fake-vomit sound you made, after you saw the cat do it for real. Looking into my mouth when I say "tun-nooool!" I laugh whenever you mimic me to a tee, the disgusted "gaadammit," or "I'm too tired!" I laugh to see your autistic strut to some inner music, on your toes jaunty-bouncy. I laugh because you like to touch dolls' ears to your eyelashes. Because you take the longest baths in history. And for all the hilarious things you say, clearly meaningful in your mind: "Walk in the ceiling!" "Poop computer at the carnival!" "Goddess get a watermelon!"

Moonlit slumbers

Steadily Nina gains more ease with the world—and bedtime is one more hurdle cleared. When Kai hoists his footrest at night and leans back on the La-Z-Boy, I lie down beside Nina. Even though I must still be at her side as she prepares to make the nightlong journey, at least now she will stay there until morning without me. Her eight years of waking periodically, sometimes screaming, sometimes laughing, were thankfully ended by one simple nutrient, B6, that allows everyone peace until dawn. On the nutrient path, gratitude happens.

After singing a lullaby I track my breath, in and out, waiting for a big vision, a spiritual pat on the back for all I've been through. Monotony substitutes for patience while my daughter continues kicking, peeping, or smacking a stuffed animal. Thus I recline in Nina's room as long as she needs me, listening as she pops her lips in a precise rhythm that punctuates the air-cleaner's whirr. "Mom stay!" she orders, if I so much as wiggle for a little more space.

And it is mystical enough to lie still in a dark room where a child settles down to dream, especially when the moon is traveling the length of the skylight notched in the ceiling. Finally little snores arise among the soft feathers of her breathing, signaling only minutes to go before I may slide off the thin edge of mattress I've been given next to Brown Horse, Green Frog. Both started out on top of her, as if she can only fall asleep with her face shielded from the night.

Moonlight makes the rational mind waver here among the walls' Spartan rectangles, and again my thoughts play on. If only she could have an ordinary girl's room, decorated by herself as an ordinary girl. Posters and framed pictures of fairies and princesses never hang on these walls. Nina is a tactile creature and keen for the sounds of things. Decorations are ripped or dismantled because it's her way of searching out their essence, gaining an intimacy with objects. Studious, almost meditative, she explores destruction. The snap of conquered wood, the nails-on-chalkboard sounds of torn, slick paper somehow serve to orient her.

Once Nina sinks deep I roll out of bed with one hand to the floor, a leg over the side, practicing the most stealth these middle-aged bones can muster. I take a last look at her room in the moonlight. Could I try some fabric art in here? Something like jute, strong and silent, unfriendly to small hands? Would a warm piney wainscoting cover up the damage she's already done, perhaps deflect her from flicking more paint off the sheetrock, hold up against her heels' attack on the walls?

So it really is about appearances, then. Why does a girly room mean so much to me, when Nina could care less? Too often, too easily, things slide from being about Nina to being about me.

But because Nina still develops, however slow or idiosyncratically, we still give her aid. We will open all channels to potential healing, and we—Kai and I—will hold onto each other. We may be in love still, beneath that ever-present monster known as *stress*, beneath change.

This is no time for anyone to give up on the other.

An incorrect dread: Nina's approaching puberty

Someday Nina will be a woman. The thought frightens me.

What mother doesn't think of it with mixed emotions? A feminist might dream of it this way: *I hope you have it better than I did. Be stronger, stand taller, and don't make excuses for yourself.* Maybe, secretly: *Wait as long as you can to become a mother.*

A woman who claims to have loved the Goddess should wax in the most positive vein. *Menses—the sacred blood of life! Motherhood—the essential spiritual epiphany!*

I'm speaking as a woman who never got to feel my belly swell with that mystery of all mysteries. Instead, I was handed a child who demanded an act of redemption. What of this girl who gets the help but is not yet healed?

What will I say to my daughter with autism? How do I explain the seep of monthly blood from between her legs, the growing poke of breasts out of her favorite kitty shirt, the urge to grab a body, which will no doubt in her case qualify as *inappropriate* to say the least?

Books, that's it. We'll get books that explain. Oh darn, those texts are all way above her nonexistent reading level. Where are the picture books? Anatomy—okay. But how will I convey it, the fallopian spread, the uterine well…*this is in your tummy…*? I'll have to leave out the scary punch line: *it's so you can make your own baby someday!* Happy smile, hugs, female bonding, visions of grandchildren—oh, wait, that's for someone else's daughter.

Knowing that what we have done to the Earth is rebounding on our health, our minds, our human future somehow pushes my grief beyond Nina's lost quality of life to the very boundaries of human existence. I can't get the *why, why, why?* out of my head.

Give up madness

Even with the mental health profession floundering, failing to staunch the spread of bona fide chronic stress, disease, and pain, we still resist the nutrient approach. It's about more than Pharma derailing that option with its expensive campaigns, isn't it?

Inroads have been made. Alternative medicine for diseases of the body is an acceptable business now. A parallel universe, perhaps, but tolerated. Yet why do we say the mentally ill will always be with us? Do we *need* them to be sick?

The double-sided coin on which genius gleams "heads!" (and the worn lunatic reads "tails!") is seductive. It promises something can be redeemed from the anguish. Like the yin-yang symbol, there's a speck of the other in each, light and shadow spinning in circular embrace. Genius-madness is a tale of how one might triumph, if one could but break through to the other side—and live to tell. The lure of madness as creativity is a juicy carrot on a stick.

Nina has no access to the weapons my brothers and I used to save ourselves. When Sam turned away from me as a child, he thought I was letting him down when I didn't share his passion for the theory of relativity. Passing me off as just a dumb girl was his trial run at a new weapon called contempt, but it got the better of him. Before long he regarded everyone from inside his armor. He knew he was, as our parents always drilled into us, *smarter than the average bear.* But not in the way our literary father hoped.

Artists and writers are the premier examples of the price we accept must be paid for the gifts of the muse. Their tragedies seem to promote the angel-demon wrestle inside creative minds. The literary names my father taught in lit classes are still revered. Sylvia Plath, Robert Lowell, Virginia Woolf, Randall Jarrell, Ann Sexton, Theodore Roethke, F. Scott Fitzgerald—all victims of the blackest moods, some dead by their own hands. Poets and storytellers, they are throwbacks to an earlier age of oral tradition, when bards were shamans and mystics too. Their rhythms inspire us, and if they must dip into madness to sing, we accept their depression as a necessary component. Would they want to rid themselves of their illness if they could?

No matter, for the genius can hoist himself up from the depths for our edification. The problem is, it's a Horatio Alger story. Pull yourself up by your bootstraps. It's all about, and only about, marshaling the necessary sheer will and strength of character to reach the masterpiece. Or, in the case of some celebrated artists, the fog one day simply dissipates. How scientific! And if one's not lucky enough to bear up until the spontaneous "lift," pass the drugs, please.

If the creative mind is sentenced to go mad and then regain its bearings willy-nilly, who wants to risk creativity? Hence we have an idolized few willing to gamble on beating the reaper. Contrast this model with Julia Cameron's *The Artist's Way*, an immensely popular self-help book that reassures the artist within us all about the inner child, about abundance, strength, and self-love. Cameron's healing syllabus for the recovery of repressed creativity produces art—through health and self-esteem. One need not be tormented or inebriated to engage the muses. Remember, too, that ancient and (pre-colonized) Native art explored nature without the need for conflict and angst.

True, not everyone's an artist or even reads—a great many are touched only by television and computer graphics. Yet all walks of life still cling to the construct of "mental illness." Why assume it's ethical to pour wealth and brainpower into the cure for cancer or AIDS, while leaving the most stranded minds—the autistic—at the rock bottom of the list? Even Pharma, which should be most keen on a cure, knows that at best it merely manages symptoms.

Could it be because the Other is always necessary to sop up our projections, to personify evil? The Other: a dumping ground for those human traits and tendencies that don't belong within the refinements of religion, civic-mindedness, art, business, happy family. The Other: a person who evokes extreme discomfort. Some call our distancing from the Other a maneuver that allows us to run from our own shadow, the disenfranchised aspects of self we abhor.

Fear of the Other may be a hard-wired human need, flaring in the interests of protection. But how far does it go? Woman as Other. Dark-skinned as Other. When mind is the crown of creation, the loss of one's mind signals failure—and failures, in a Type A society, are the worst Others imaginable. Who wants to see the brain defiled by crazy people, hyperactive or nonverbal kids, criminals, the weird? We prefer they be good (silent) and go get their (limited) help. There is many a pill for the infinite variations on the Other.

And it's always profitable, for someone, if there is an Other you are loath to become. Fearful individuals buy products and services to safeguard against the slide into Otherness. Pharma feeds Otherness with platitudes about getting help. "Help," also known as a band-aid on a boo-boo, won't cut it when the sorrows, the behaviors, the debilitating toxic load on damaged minds change human beings beyond reversal.

I couldn't "help" Diana the caregiver, surrogate target for the help I needed to give my brother Sam.

I want more than "help" for Nina, though I acknowledge that Sam's time for help may have run out. As a mother—and someone who almost fell into the jaws of perpetual "help" as a teenager—I can't give up on my little messenger now. Nina belongs to a segment of our future that will require special services and medicine for a long, budget-straining time to come. What happens when the depressed, toxic, wordless, and anxious among us become the majority?

These are heavy troubles to hold. So I tried to think like a scientist. The resistance to giving up madness seemed like a stubborn virus, but in order to locate an antidote I needed to know more about where such resistance came from. The *why?* has morphed into *where from?* Like scientists who are stuck and then stumble on an answer in a dream, I asked for a picture, an image that might help me track the source, the root, the repeating mandate that started somewhere and was pervasively deployed. *Where did we get this need for the Other (worthless evil) and the conviction that what is good may only arise from suffering?*

In reply, a childhood memory surfaced. Within the recessed, lit alcove of the dark hallway at the Finley farm, a statue of Jesus tore at his bleeding heart.

Chapter 21
THE VITAL SHE

Walking the land wasn't enough to unwind a body aging its way into a stressful menopause. Most of the women I knew had grandchildren already (and a tacit agreement with life to slow down) while I was still dealing with a toilet-training problem that might never resolve. Nutrients had pulled my thoughts and energy out of the trash bin, but I'd ignored the rest of me. Years of fight-or-flight readiness had twisted this neck, shoulders, and back into knots.

Finally, there were signs I could begin to relax. Nina seemed well on her way down the biomedical trail. "Biomed moms" is shorthand for those of us who view autism as a serious environmental mishap, rather than a mysterious flick of the genes. Biomed is not confined to natural alternatives in medicine, but mothers often end up there after picking and choosing among pharmaceuticals with care. We lean away from putting more toxins into our children, although the spectrum of some parents' choices does include antidepressants and antipsychotics. There is nothing I can do about keeping such company. For now, it's better to have those who are seeking and learning on board, even if they aren't yet ready to give up the dream of a miracle drug.

Many pursue another avenue on the quest: educational advances, particularly behavioral therapy. These one-on-one methods of learning can bring a child into a gamut of further skills. Not all parents who embrace behaviorism are biomed, but most biomed moms are a thorn in the side of their local Special Education services, pushing for techniques that do more than help a special needs child pass the time.

Kai and I finally persuaded our school district to employ a consultant with the skills of Applied Behavioral Analysis (ABA). Things come slower to the heartland, but after intensive training of staff and a six-inch thick notebook of data sheets and instructions to guide her day,

Nina was finally getting somewhere in school. I was pleased as punch and exhaling some overdue sighs of relief.

But what of the frame that encompassed this middle-aged, adoptive biomed mother with a Pagan past and yearnings to feel the spirit stir? The nutrients I took in each day—minerals and vitamins, herbs, green superfoods, and an allergen-free diet—worked to regain my mind and to propel my energy into the warrior mode. I'd lost and kept off the weight that gluten, dairy, and four miscarriages had pounded on, yet I remained out of touch with the rest of the flesh, this bony carriage and all the connective tissue that worked to maintain the pace required for raising Nina. I thought back fondly to the days when I did yoga; maybe I'd start again. But first I needed something like a nurturing jackhammer to break down the barriers. Massage was once a regular event before children. I needed it even more now.

Male massage therapists were plentiful in Osage End, but now I was shy. Was it because I was older? Probably. Married? Kai did have a jealous streak. Or was there also an urge to make a ceremonial re-entry into a new phase, and my choice of therapist needed to further the plan of mindfulness throughout the experience?

A business card in the health-food market advertised a female massage therapist who worked only on women. A good gamble, if not the perfect solution.

So it was that I arrived at a weathered bungalow in Osage End's historic neighborhood, where a tall, strong-looking Amazon answered the door. Clearly, she could put the moves on muscles of steel. The massage space was a spare bedroom in her home; hardwood floors gleamed as we passed the kitchen where garden tomatoes crowded the sink. Rose was twenty-five years old, her son away at preschool as clients arrived for quiet and peace.

Massage rooms and clutter don't mix, so every decoration counts. In Rose's room the pregnant-goddess art could have been nothing more than affirmations of birth, since she did prominently market her prenatal massage skills. Turning over under smooth sheets after having my back unwound, I looked around at the big mamas surrounded by the cycles of the moon, at prehistoric belly-wisdom beauties carved in vanilla-scented soap. "So," I pointed and smiled, "these are interesting."

"A friend supplies me with this art," she said. She was hesitant but something lingered in the air, an invitation to say more.

"There's a lot to be said for letting women's bodies into spiritual iconography," I replied.

"I grew up in a fundamentalist Christian church. It was…a different world than in here," ventured Rose.

I snorted and mentioned my Catholic girlhood. "Most of those homes have pictures of Jesus and crucifixes on the wall. I like it better in here." I sighed as Rose dug into a spot on my upper back that was a bull's eye for tension release.

I drifted into silence under her hands, and once again saw the long hallway at the Finleys that cut the farmhouse in two. You entered it from the dining room, the lively scene of holiday dinners around the long table and at card tables where the youngest ones sat. You always shut the door behind you, for the hall was dark and still as a sepulcher. With bedrooms at either end with doors always closed, and more closed doors leading to another bedroom and the bathroom, the hall was silent and private.

When my cousins and I were little we'd sometimes throw on the light and run, sliding in our socks down the hall's length. But that was rare, for the corridor's inviolate darkness and shush seemed an intrinsic part of the house. One left the sunny commonality of family reunions to navigate the hall by dim light peeking out from under the doors. And by the Jesus alcove, although most of the time the little nightlight was burned out. Lit or not, you knew he was there, oversized heart leaping from his chest. I couldn't look. As a child it seemed too scary, like the huge statues in church. Later, I developed unease about the heart muscle. Hearts equaled cardiology and you-know-who. Funny, how your mind can weave all over the place during a massage.

Rose emerged from some reflections of her own. "Ah, Jesus. What to do about him? Once I got out of the church, I took a hard look at it all. I knew there had to be another point of view. When I came across good evidence that Jesus was married, I flipped out. Excited, thrilled, blown away—I wanted to go up to perfect strangers and say, 'Hey folks, Jesus was married to Mary Magdalene!'"

My eyes flew open. "Really? To the prostitute?" This was a new one on me.

"Only she wasn't. Early Christians knew it," Rose said. "I mean, *early* early Christians." After a few more lamentations about how much her former community would disapprove, my masseuse shared the questions on her mind.

"If the two of them were married and she was no prostitute, what was their mission? I'm thinking there's more about this Jesus we weren't told. If people of his time really believed Jesus *was* God, what did that make his beloved? Reverse it: if Mary Magdalene *wasn't* a goddess, what did that make her husband?"

"Now you are really messing with my mind," I murmured. Frankly, I felt a yawn coming on, an urge to fall asleep on the table, but one thing kept me awake: the quality of Rose's interest in the topic combined with the proudly female imagery in this room, at once a place of business and an expression of her deeper self. The Goddess was being re-translated here.

Rose was more than just a recovering fundamentalist; neither did she fit the Neo-Pagan type I remembered so well. Clearly her first love was healing, but spirituality was also on the tip of her mind. She wanted me to know she was onto something, and apparently there was an explosion of research, bursting into popular view in the form of everything from novels to nonfiction bestsellers. It sounded like a unique Christian inquiry that challenged the picture I'd been fed in catechism classes. I was getting a lot more than a rubdown here.

But I resisted out of more than just my urge to snooze. Frankly, it was my prejudice. What would this mean to Pagans who staked their identity on opposition to Christianity? Ouch—I was still in sympathy with the likes of them.

Leaving Rose's house floating on air, with the major kinks loosened from my shoulders, I thought about Mary Magdalene. I balked at the idea of a goddess in Christianity, unable to trust that a Father God would make Her any more than a "helpmate." But Rose talked about the Gnostic gospels, those lost-then-recently-found books that never made it into the Bible, and how they told a different story. The discovery of these Gnostic gospels in an urn buried under the sands of Egypt—and the widely read commentary by Elaine Pagels—had ushered in ideas out of sync with the standard Jesus tale.

I felt as though I'd been out of the loop in more ways than one. I'd missed this interest in a Christian goddess while sticking to the shores of science. How refreshing to think about something else for a change!

At my next massage, I learned more about Pagels' work. The question had been bugging me—how did the Gnostics get away with it? "For one thing," Rose said, "the way I read it is that after Jesus walked and talked, there were Christians with all kinds of practices and beliefs. Very diverse. Like using the term 'New Age'—what exactly does that mean? A whole host of things, but you know what it is when you're around it. I guess Gnostics were like that—you could spot 'em, and the official church eventually did a lot more than just complain about 'em. "

"What about hatred of the flesh? That seems a Christian trademark, no matter who's preaching." I figured this point would interest a bodyworker.

"Some Gnostics were downright tantric," Rose grinned. "You know, sexual magic. They really only had one thing in common: diversity! Hey, haven't you met New Agers out of touch with their bodies, too? All ether and no Earth? But there was one large tract of common ground in the Gnostic past. They all held dear the pursuit of a direct, no-middleman pipeline to the divine called gnosis, or self-knowledge."

At this point, I asked for a light blanket over the one-sheet drape. Rose kept the room on the cool side. "These old houses are a bear to heat!" she sighed.

"And I suppose women were given free rein to just…be?"

"Pretty much. The equality of women, spiritual leaders in their own rights—a matter of course when Mother God stands equal to the Father."

"What was their name for," I cleared my throat, "the Goddess?"

Rose didn't miss a beat. "Most people, if they know about Gnostics, think of Sophia. But the Gnostics had many names for the divine feminine. Let me see…Grace…Silence…The Womb…Mother of the

All. There were some others. Wisdom, Thought, and some pretty high-brow terms like Intelligence, Foresight. I call her the Divine Feminine."

Sounded like the Goddess to me. Rose finished off my feet with a flourish, and as I sighed deeply she imparted something else that sounded familiar. In Gnosticism the "divine feminine" was the Source; Yahweh was Her consort, who tended to get uppity and power-mad. I recalled mythologies from the same era and geographic region that showcased a divine couple in a similar tussle.

During my next appointment I told Rose about my forays with Cedar Wing and the local Earth-lovers in the days long before Nina. Over the weeks I hopped on and off her table, I read some Gnostic fragments and the commentary by Pagels, slowly losing the frozen resentment and fear about anything resembling my Catholic schooling. I was fascinated by the possibility of Her presence getting more airplay through Christianity, of all places! I doubted I would ever be one to go gaga for Mary Magdalene, but to contemplate this aspect of the Goddess' universality—well, it gave me hope for the world.

Still, wariness of Jesus was wrapped up with the Inquisitor-fear. Long hair and a beard weren't enough to make me overlook the biblical insistence on Father, Father, and Father. Thinking of him as married to a powerful woman did iron out some of the wrinkles, though.

Rose was a new breed. She wasn't the Inquisition-fearing, oppositional Pagan of my bygone boot camp days. She saw a mesh between the Divine Feminine, as she called it, and the Goddess, as I had known Her. After one particularly great massage, she mentioned that a group of women with similar inclinations toward the female divine met regularly, talking and sharing food. They were not sure how to proceed beyond that. Would I come guide them into ritual?

And now for something more…normal?

In no time at all I found myself teaching again, having the time of my life sharing magic as if every wish had always come true, guiding these women toward their guides when mine were silent, creating sacred space as if there were no rift between Her and me. How did this happen?

Because the women were young, they were eager and they asked. Maybe I thought some of it would rub off. Perhaps, although mindfulness and the example of the Buddha were near and dear additions to my limited array of coping mechanisms, I simply needed Mom.

There was another kind of synergy among us. I talked about Nina every time we socialized, both before and after our focused work, and these women were up on what seemed to be happening to children these days. None of them had a diagnosed child, but they all knew a parent from preschool or a day care center who was grappling with a behavioral disorder or developmental disability. The women knew the autism epidemic was growing. They were all ears about the dietary and detox interventions we'd done with Nina. It was a sign of the times.

A friend who'd known me since the village-witch days volunteered her living room for our meetings. Couches and plants were pushed against one wall to make a cozy space for six twenty-somethings, plus one mother pushing fifty who took the floor. Our hostess brewed herbal concoctions that we downed by the mug as the young women discussed their fears, the detractors among their husbands, and the Christian majority. It seemed like not *that* much had really changed.

We dotted the room with candles. In the center of our crosslegged circling, on a piece of board covered by a shimmering cloth, were our tools. Incense for the element of air, one tall candle for laughing fire, a chalice of pure water, and stones of all colors, polished and rough. A figurine I'd dusted off from my collection: Isis, the magical, medicinal mother, the first savior, She whose husband's death and rebirth prefigured the Christian Resurrection. Isis devotees still existed, bearing many versions of that story, at the time when all types of Gnostics peopled the Mediterranean and Near East.

Just like the old days, we'd close our eyes in order to "ground," sinking visualized roots toward the earth, turning to the directions to call them near. Then the work. Work of air, crafting pictures of mind to make goals manifest. Work of fire, raising the power as a cone that sails to destinations of desire. Work of water, learning to feel, heeding the night-dreams. Work of earth, making medicine bags of herb and stone to carry and remind us of the pledge to be authentic, empowered, Earth-wise.

If I'd supposedly turned my back on magic, why was it so much fun? Why was it, throughout our weeks in that little living room, so meaningful and spirit-connected?

Too long an isolated parent, it was good for me to get out of the house. Even though I didn't care for the use of "divine" in tandem with the word "feminine" (once synonymous with ladylike), there was an excitement of change that was hard to resist. The Goddess, under any description, would never be ladylike. But maybe the Inquisition was not a foregone conclusion the moment Jesus of Nazareth embarked with his plan. She had been there all along in his day, the one he called, in *The Gospel to the Hebrews*, "My Mother, the Spirit."

Here was a surprise chance for reconciliation between Pagans and Christians. Who could have imagined such news would prompt the Goddess to set me ticking again?

Moonspeak returns

Whenever Nina takes a bath, our deck is the place to catch moonrise. I put my feet up, scanning the curves of wooded hills that contradict notions of Kansas as flat and boring. Waiting for the moon, I'll weave along the railing some tendrils of wisteria surging forth. Twilight blots out the power lines where bluebirds and green hummers perch by day.

I still make a wish on the first star as sunset's final purple ribbon turns to gray. I can't always stay for the rise of a full moon, but lately I've re-committed to the practice. It's all part of the return of the Goddess to my heart.

I'd never made a break, never denounced—how silly, as if She would care!—the female face of God. But I did scratch magic, ritual, and moon talks off my list. I crafted my tragedy and transformation as a trial that unseen forces had meted out. On bad days it was punishment, while on better days the Nina saga was a lesson and a revelation. I still hoped that clear, positive thoughts about the future could make it so. Affirmations were a form of quick hypnosis, since trance no longer produced guides more real to me than neighbors and kin.

Mindfulness was a helpful rescue technique. But as for living in the present, I could scarcely give up scheming on strategies for Nina's recovery.

Yet something happened, after so many years of effort. I looked out from autism toward the world, and by mutual consent She emerged as never before. Now, my place to greet Her is more comfortable than a rough hay bale rolled round, but She and I talk once again. It's only a little like the time when Her radiant face topped my post-divorce house in the Flint Hills. The difference is that supplication is replaced by gratitude.

A package heal

How can anyone whose options turned out like mine and Kai's have room for gratitude? At first I was wary of brainwashing myself with perky platitudes. But She was back, Nina was gaining, and if magic taught me anything, it's that the mind's orientation creates the world.

Many nights, as the moon slinks up the eastern sky, I'll craft a mental gratitude list whose number one heading is *health*. Of mind: no more anxious, paranoid thoughts, no more sabotage of intimate relationships. Of body: migraine-free, I can exercise, enjoy food, maintain energy and my immune system. I take no prescription medication.

But how does one pick nutrients for the spiritual path? What works for me is to journal, walk the woods and prairie, circle with sisters in the ceremonies we create. One of the beauties of these new, alternative spiritualities is the permission to create our own traditions. Realizing that prayer can take any form, in any venue, at any moment, it also helps to know that others have walked their unique ways before us.

There for the taking is a lineage more profound than any one individual's environmentally spawned, family disease. People once knew how to treat delusions and depressions, but we have forgotten. Forgotten that we had foremothers and forefathers who used plant medicine and foods to heal, who praised the natural elements and freely gave wise counsel in the bosom of true community. The best of them were slandered and suppressed, once their vibrant, vital Mother's body was construed as little more than sinful dirt. I imagine these forebears are urging on those of us who can still think and stay calm, urging us to listen to messengers like Nina. The way I see it, she is these ancestors' gift to me.

How could I have borne it if I had never tread by accident upon the environmental roots of the malaise that claimed Sam and clipped Nina's wings? And what would life have been like without her, the blue-eyed beauty, the catalyst whose suffering seized my cherished notions, shredded and recast them? How would I ever have stopped running from the memory of the Habitat, the specter of the mind-thrashing family disease?

Might I have become one of those legal clients Kai represents, the ones whose migraine syndromes justify monthly payments of rightful disability benefits, with a trail of medical records to tell the story and days of painful stumbling from one doozy of a headache to another? Unable to work, unable to play, unable to serve a single good cause in the world? Overcome by chronic pain that misshapes thoughts into self-loathing?

Or would I have joined Sam on the drug-train to complicating side effects? Wouldn't I have accepted it as fact—finally succumbing without protest to the only known explanation of events beyond my control—that the Wohler Madness could not be cured?

How, without Nina, would I have seen through Sam's disgrace? How, without her inability to feel any relief from Pharma's wares (seizure meds, antibiotics, anti-inflammatories) could questions addressed to the supreme medical authorities have formed in this mind? Without her, how would I have forgiven my brother for his contempt when he was the best brain, the smartest bear of us all? Would I have allowed myself to realize it was all such a waste—the demise of Sam's future, the uncertainty of Nina's, perhaps even my infertility—and all so unnecessary?

Whether or not I can ever tell Nina about the perils of patriarchy and the good parts about living free in spite of it, she is female. I'm left to wonder whether a culture in which females hold the reins of healing alongside their male counterparts would ever allow autism. Nina reminds me of these kinds of questions every day. After her bath she will trail out here to say goodnight to the moon, making us a private triptych: the eternal, the mother, the maiden…moon, middle-ager, autistic. We are one.

Gratitude for knowledge—gnosis—is my reward, albeit laced with sorrow for the ones you try and try to save, but can't. Gratitude infiltrates body, mind, and spirit, making fertile ground for insight.

Isn't that plenty? But there was more. The moon would open me to an even wider vision. I thought a view of autism as a harbinger of worsening environmental plague was all I could hold. I was wrong.

Tough lunar love

The week had been hot for May, making the atmosphere reflect a moon huge and nearly crimson. Such a sight was already enough to shift awareness up a notch, but while I was in a light rapture She took advantage. That voice, The Great Within and Without, laid one more on me: *Why couldn't we abolish, eradicate, and finally retire the experience and the concept of "mental illness," once and for all?*

What a sly Divine Mother, sneaking this in at the end of my tiring day! Bowling me over and waiting to see what next. Or was the thought brewing for some time? It was the word choice that surprised me.

Abolish mental illness. That word stuck, bold and on the mark. It went beyond *cure*, though that would be the effect. The word *abolish* had a sort of antebellum ring to it. I thought of the legacy of this prairie ground as "bleeding Kansas," a state torn during the Civil War over the issue of slavery. What a fitting place to launch a new era of abolition! Abolish the authoritarian rule of the diagnosis with its mandatory drug-daze inside our minds, taking down the body bit by bit.

To abolish mental illness would mean to give up the madness-genius temptation—give up the need for the totally-out-of-it Other, give up our addiction to calling *crazy* that which we do not *as yet* understand. What was it Friedrich Wohler said, in another context, about "things unknown?"

But we shall learn to know them. The irony wouldn't escape Wohler that what we must now come to know is a sensibility about wholeness and nature that was the norm in his day, although fading fast to the tune of the industrial age.

Letting go of the famous scientist continued to be a gift. I could set sail without dragging that anchor I both loved and loathed to drop. I was also free from resentment about his frequent mercury-handlings (common in that day for chemists) and imagining who knows what other toxin may have snuck into his DNA, poisoning every descendant right down to me. At last, only an average bear, the freedom from pressure paradoxically encouraged a deeper and wider view of what was shaping up to be my mission.

I recalled the first time I spoke with the Moon. Her message was pointed directly at my circumstances; it was a life raft, a sea change offered by the tide-puller that She is. This time, I heard her thinking of the entire world—without forgetting Nina or the new diagnoses and drug prescriptions dished out daily across that world.

The environmental crisis has become extremely personal. Cleaning up our mess means more than protecting waters, skies, trees, and soil—we are among the endangered as well. We are not merely a cancerous growth deserving of extinction because we spoiled our own biosphere. After all, did we know every step of the way what would be the consequences? Were we at best only naïve? Did the likes of Wohler ever think ahead and shudder over possibilities, or did he simply rejoice, a nature lover suddenly able to mimic Mom?

Wohler invested in a nickel mine. Nickel, now a known carcinogen, was one of those metals I watched for on those lab sheets that told us what was coming out of Nina's body. Did he ever suspect its not-so-silver lining? Today, all of Europe regulates how much nickel is allowed in products that come in contact with human skin. Meanwhile, sophisticated campaigns convince the public that plastic is just fine, food additives do no harm, and warming weather trends are merely seasonal. Will we ever make up our minds now that we know too much—not gnosis but information, so much information that, without gnosis, sorting it out is a chore?

Wohler's kind was in pursuit of a heady rush toward gnosis. Too bad it was only partial. After the Inquisition erased women's holistic medical knowledge, privatized the common areas that fed folk with foraging and game, and quelled "superstitious" Earth-loving religious practices, the chemical quest became a Father God game that would pay for erasing the vital force, "Our Mother, the Spirit."

What if it's too late? What if there is too much invested, and damaged minds are only capable of going for immediate gratification? Thank the many stars there are persons left with the emotional intelligence to walk the most direct—and ethical—path to healing. I find them in those who uphold the value of body and mind living free of unseen poisons, so we might get back on the evolutionary trek. To know—all of it. Gnosis, complete, but a knowledge as yet still hidden. To search for real health of person and planet today is not only revolutionary, it is the path of enlightenment.

These are the ideas that the Moon, rising through the Earth's umbra, spoke to my conscience. When I sensed that the lesson was done—Nina was yelling for mom—I ran back inside. Before grabbing a towel, I searched for a moving passage in *Our Stolen Future: A Medical Detective Story*:

> Some might find irony in the prospect that humans in their restless quest for dominance over nature may be inadvertently undermining their own ability to reproduce or to learn and think. They may see poetic justice in the possibility that we have become unwitting guinea pigs in our own vast experiment with synthetic chemicals. But in the end, it is hard to regard such a chemical assault on our children and their potential for a full life as anything but profoundly sad. Chemicals that disrupt [the body's innate biochemical] messages have the power to rob us of rich possibilities that have been the legacy of our species and, indeed, the essence of our humanity. There may be fates worse than extinction.

Still waiting for a happy ending

Nina is twelve. Nina has not recovered from autism.

Nina speaks not, plays not, learns not, eats not—a *lot* not—like other children. Our family was supposed to be elsewhere by now, our anguish packed up and put out with the trash.

Now that she is past the all-important age for "early intervention," I get the feeling I'm supposed to calm down and bear up, slow down the search for what ails her and quit trying to make the puzzle pieces fit. I get this message from the special education professionals who adore her, but still harbor the low expectations they are required by law to put in writing. I get this from the doctors who are not too ashamed to throw up their hands. I wonder sometimes if I'm seeing it in Kai, in his resistance to trying a new treatment.

Am I supposed to sit with others of my kind who have likewise *learned to live with it* and to become silent observers of the so-called normal world? To be told I'm a saint for parenting such a special child, and then dutifully put one step ahead of the other day after day into eternity, until Nina, Kai, and I are dead ashes?

There is also the more difficult—and more insulting—challenge to believe that before conception Nina somehow chose this earthwalk knowing full well what was coming: the lifelong struggle to perceive persons and events through veils of pain. If only I could just say that *the autistic will always be with us.*

But wouldn't I be missing Her voice, the Earth who might possibly be using this disorder to yell at humankind, "Wake up! Look out!"?

Thus Nina turns out to be a chosen child of Goddess after all.

But as she ages from tender toward teenaged, I sense a change in outsiders' graciousness and empathy. Said a woman to me the other day, "You've got to let her live her own life," which at the time I found somewhat cold. I struggle to see the truth-kernel: what if the soul that became Nina considered taking this on, back there in some spirit world where she waited for another chance to bloom in the flesh? Sound too far-fetched, too metaphysical? Even quantum physics challenges the notion of linear time. Why would Nina, or any soul, volunteer if not out of a great altruism, a willingness to give up grappling for the goodies and dedicate the next life instead to service? The messenger as message. Thank Goddess that Nina found someone who, on occasion, is faith-full enough to see her for the fine missionary she is. I will always love her for picking me.

There was a time when I'd enter Nina's room in the morning wishing she might have passed peacefully back to that other world in her sleep. Goddess, forgive me! Now the opposite understanding dawns: if she were not, I would stand bereft. What she endures for the sins committed against the Earth is a sign of a remarkable spirit. It is my privilege to attend her suffering and make her feel as comfortable, as loved, as I can.

And because the Goddess *is* the world—assailed by horrors like mercury, yes, but still adorned with prairie flowers and azure seas—I can't play the petulant child with Her any more than I can close the quest for Nina, sequestered inside her "disorder." *They are one and the same.*

New heretics for Her

Here is one way to view the parent-driven nature of autism research, in which moms and dads are so often cast as shrill and simplistic. This view encompasses the mothers in mental-health advocacy groups who are also organizing, standing up as mothers for the sons and daughters the system ensnares.

Females, with nowhere to go but back to the home to manage our outcast children (a full-time job), predominate in today's quest for gnosis about body and mind. This sexist situation backfires because these mothers are mad as hell. Whether or not they "believe" in the female Divine, they embody the Mother who will be firm and persistent in protecting her own. These parents, family members, or faithful friends fly under radar with research from the world of functional, or integrative medicine and congregate on computer listserves to exchange knowledge. Yet often solitary in their own communities, they manage a deep breath before begging a scornful M.D. to take a tiny risk on nutrients. These new Gnostics may be praying in the strictest of Father-God churches on Sunday, but like it or not, they go forth as an embodiment of the Divine Mother. In contrast to Creator stands the *Creatrix* whose way is not to demand obedience, but rather to offer the gorgeous world and ask only simple respect in return. Will Her ways ever become "organized religion?" I hope not.

In this world the best of humanity is tracking real justice and healing, despite the façade of a greed so amoral that it pumps mercury into a pregnant womb (flu shots, still laced with the stuff). Parents of suffering offspring have no problem with saying we must cure, we must defeat, we must do away with autism. We've pulled it off—we have "reframed" the disorder. It's still a struggle, but we do not fear envisioning, implementing, and seeking knowledge again.

Yet few seem ready to give up the great dumping ground of madness, so tragic, even horrific, but potentially delicious to those outside. Even to some wearing the label, losing it would mean that there is nowhere to go but conformity and consumerism. But giving up the need for Others assumed to have lost their minds really means abandoning the lexicon of the Helpers in order to call slow poisoning what it is. It means not giving up on the Earth, on ourselves. It means to *abolish* mental illness.

The Goddess does not evangelize

Last night at the ritual, a young mother whose Christian fundamentalist husband gives her trouble about attending said something like this: "I wish he'd understand! The Goddess is everywhere, everything! I don't care if you call Her the Female Divine, the Divine Feminine, or She of Ten Thousand Names. Call Her a new name that speaks to you. For heaven's sake, there's not a whole lot she's not, right?"

Rose chimed in. "She's been seen from the beginning as one who changes, just like we do. As a girl She is sacred, as mama She is sacred, as elder She's no less. The first 'holy trinity,' it seems to me. How anybody makes a place for Her is hardly about dogma or creed. I told my husband that *She* is Nature. Tell yours to 'step outside if you need a bible, dude!'"

The way these women treated their little girls to goddess tales and rituals made me wonder if I could be more proactive with Nina. But first, I needed to formally introduce the two.

At an altar in a small loft where Nina can't climb, I spread out a cloth and place on it cherished items, naming sacred what is sacred to me. Rigid rules fade when there's nothing to evangelize about, which is why the Goddess comes at no price. She can be an image of gender equality and never a toe in mystic waters touch. She can be a daring, inclusive thought that comes every time you hear "God, He." She can be an interesting historical study, a private dream of ecotopia if we happen to tend toward the visionary. Or She can be symbolized by statues of goddesses like caregivers attending a photo of your loved one for whom you walk the nutrient path.

On my altar to the Goddess sits a picture worth a thousand words. It is a snapshot of Nina on a school field trip. A museum exhibit calls to her and Nina leans to look intently at the display. Whatever captures her attention is outside the frame. It is the look on her sweet face in profile, the curiosity plain in the tip of her head, the straining of her bones against the railing that brings this photo to my altar. It's more than *she looks like a normal kid*; something whispers of promise.

Along the upper edge of this snapshot I place a twelve-inch high replica of the Great Mother whose religion, in the ancient world, rivaled Christianity. Isis, First Lady of Healing on a golden throne, nurses Horus the baby king. Beside Her to the east is Kuan Yin, Asian goddess of compassion and the protectress of children, smiling benignly. One by one the statues circle around, mostly mothers but also others.

The Virgin of Guadalupe, looking out for the oppressed.

Oya, the changeable wind, African mother whose children are the eight tributaries of the Niger River, suckling her newborn.

Artemis of the wild, the eternal, natural girl who came to her mother's aid as midwife at her brother's birth.

Lakshmi, the golden and chaste Indian goddess, for a wealth of happiness. (Some extra coinage for Nina's needs would also be nice.)

And, for the wise old crone, a framed picture of Georgia O'Keefe, honorary goddess.

All of them are connected by story to other names, traits, eras. They morph, they magick, they endure.

Nina, looking at a museum exhibit, is thus surrounded on the two-by-two-foot wooden shelf I drape and call an altar. The many minutes I spend just sitting there at the altar represent not so much a return to witchery as an embrace of the Mother and Sacred Others as the source of hope. We at once save Her memory and recognize that She will go on without our contrary ways. But I believe She roots for us. As the Inventor of Healing Ways She has bequeathed, once again, the nutrient path.

May She watch over Nina and aid her growth. May She watch over all of us.

The nutrient path

When detox is underway, when foods match what the body welcomes, when the need to supplement is protected from the tentacles of Pharma, then we can decide how the vessel of psychotherapy fits. Sifting and sorting through toxic psychologies that blame parents, praise the separation of the self, and ignore the Earth, we might even return to rituals and find our way to include community as witness to our healing. What would it be like to embrace a psychology of ceremony, of direct communion with wind, flame, waves, and rich, clean soil?

We'll fail if we latch onto healing at only one point of the triangle of body, mind, and spirit. No fair being a nutrient Nazi who scorns mystic bliss and mindful counsel! The "health food fanatic" rages in an evangelizing that cloaks a postmodern truth: in a world where so many feel they've lost the helm of their own lives, obsessions with diet and fitness afford a semblance of control. This type of evangelist can be a pain in the neck, because his moral base is weak: "Be healthy! For health's sake!" But why should we?

When we consider that we are part of Her body and that we're making Her ill (which makes us ill), then personal health equals planetary health, a spiritual imperative. She is the paradigm for a way of wellness that is empirical but safe. You don't have to "believe" in the Goddess to track this historically, to know that when value systems rest on holistic principles, She/Earth/We equal the Whole.

Wait a minute! Don't romanticize the past. People died awfully young back then.

And today is better? Living longer yet sicker, with children whose light fades younger and younger? Survival of the fittest no long applies; we live in danger of killing the Whole. Yet hearts tuned to the beauty and mystery of the Maternal Earth would logically steer all advances toward holism, toward approaches such as sustainable agriculture and nutrient therapy. We have the tools to do right.

Whither psychotherapy on the nutrient path? Will the profession carp about shirking personal responsibility, counter that we are hiding bad behavior behind vitamin deficiencies and toxic load? Will it ever let the brain rejoin the body long enough to understand that getting to the real root of each individual's malaise is a healing of both self and Earth?

Psychiatry as a science burgeoned when the Industrial Revolution gained speed, changing the world for most species. Our increasing disorders tell an unfolding tale of estrangement from Her. *Toxic earth, toxic mind.* The theologian turned "geologian" Thomas Berry says we are all autistic when it comes to the planet. Just as afflicted children appear to tune out their own mother, Western humans no longer see, hear, or feel the presence of their Mother, the natural world.

Once the I-Thou exchange of therapy embraces connection to the true state of the body, there will be no more cordoning off Spirit as a "private matter" or muddle for one's pastor to slog through. Fortunately, discourse on integrating the spiritual/religious urge into psychotherapy has already taken place. Perhaps the transpersonal approach will be more effective when Her values become part of the equation, the nourishing ethics of the nutrient path.

Careening down the toxic trail, fear and powerlessness fuel the tightening of our ranks into ever-smaller groups, a blathering about the sanctity of the family unit even as each member pursues, in separate rooms, the next byte via computer and TV. Meanwhile, hearts and minds shut down before the task of self and planetary stewardship. Pinned to lethargy and illness by heavy metals and industrial chemicals, the inability to detox intensifies with each generation. The culture of narcissism is fast becoming Planet Autism.

Imagine, instead, a mind full of connection with a natural place or formation. This love for place leading to another awakening: like a parent, this Mother we inhabit has so much to give. Ambivalence about—and unreasonable demands upon—human mothers everywhere begins to fade. Strident calls for "family first" and the fuming standoff about control of women's reproduction wither away as we widen the acceptable arena for family relations. We dismantle the Hatfield-and-McCoys mentality—our bloodline against everyone else's—when we glimpse what the Gnostics already knew: *separation* is the real illusion of this world, not a characteristic of the world itself.

May those who find solace and inspiration in Father God see the wisdom of letting Mother stand fully powerful at His side, recalling Him to Earth Spirit as well. We walk on Her flesh, our skin a piece of Hers. All matter, our alma mater, is singing and dancing and may be Her smile. I fear that we will not survive without an openness to Her return. She is the first body that nourished the vital force, creating billions of ways to show it, always wearing ten thousand names and never fighting about it. She was the vessel and the inspiration for our first spiritual longings. The vital force, released from doctrines of Vitalism that tried to name Her by what She was not. Released (soon, I hope) from synthetic substances that seek to imitate every miracle She produced before we primates even trotted the savannah. Released from the sorrowful truth that every girl and boy being born has less and less of a chance for purity, intelligence, survival.

Whether a mighty mythos to aid healthcare reform, or a voice for wholeness heard in the mind, the Divine Feminine is medicine this planet needs.

ACKNOWLEDGEMENTS

Gratitude goes to the land I named Heron's Way: the circle, Little Buck Creek, the hawks, and the hill. I am blessed by you. I also wish to thank the forest and community of Shantivanam in Easton, Kansas. Parts of this book were written on retreat there, as well as in picnic shelters at the Slough Creek Conservation District in Jefferson County, where moonrise is a spectacular event.

Many thanks to the courageous citizen's groups, practitioners and individuals who resist the drugs-for-dampening approach pushed on the minds of adults, children, the elderly, and even our pets. Thanks go especially to the far-reaching vision and persistence of Dan Stradford, founder of Safe Harbor International.

To Dr. Abram Hoffer, grandfather of a truly holistic psychiatry: selfishly I wish you had lived past your ripe old age to write the Foreword to my book, as you had so graciously consented. I cherish your encouraging e-mails to this stranger from Kansas. Smile on us from the next world!

Genita Petralli, nutritional biochemist, coined the phrase "Green Mental Healthcare." Her civic work with Green Body and Mind in Santa Cruz, California, was a model for grassroots mental wellness.

Dr. Tyler Woods, psychotherapist of the Mindhance Learning Center, facilitated my certification as a Holistic Mental Health Coach through the American Association of Drugless Practitioners (AADP). Thank you for this and for your patience.

As an editor, Laura Conner was meticulous, creative, and engaged. Victoria Foth Sherry's skills at copyediting added the final touch of inspired finesse. Denise Enck handles Web matters with an artist's eye.

Elizabeth Long worked diligently to expose the genealogical entanglements of my Wohler relations.

For many types of support and mindful critique, thanks go to Joyce and David McCullough, Barbara Neighbors Deal, Patricia Lynn Reilly, Natasha Kern, Women's Web, Donna White, Farrell Hoy Jenab, Jay Pryor, Judy and Roy Todd, Caryn Miriam-Goldberg, Dr. Stephen

Ilardi and Maria Ilardi, Cheryl Miller, Melissa Mitchell, Cindy DeGraw, Christine Garvey, Karen Foglesong, Chuck Franks, Corinna West, awesome bossman Cliff Tisdale, and all my Natural Mind students and coaching clients.

For her intelligence and caring loyalty, Angela Rocha, practically a co-parent and definitely our rock, deserves a special thank you from our family.

Gratefulness goes to my mother for upholding the values of compassion, relatedness, and civility. I wish I had not given her such a hard time for so many years.

It's often said that immediate family suffers most during a book's labor. This one was particularly difficult. For steadfastness of support and willingness to weather storms—especially when so many couples raising autistic children divorce—my husband has my deepest love and gratitude.

✳ ✳ ✳

"Even though chemists as a group..." Cathy Cobb and Harold Goldwhite, *Creations of Fire: Chemistry's Lively History from Alchemy to the Atomic Age* (Plenum Press, 1995)

"...a moral crisis that must be addressed." Robert F. Kennedy, Jr., "Deadly Immunity," Rolling Stone, June 20, 2005

"My heart is moved by all I cannot save..." Adrienne Rich, excerpted from "Natural Resources," in *The Dream of a Common Language* (Norton, 1978)

"Women who reject..." Phyllis Chesler, *Women and Madness*, (Palgrave MacMillan, 2005)

"Some might find irony in the prospect that humans..." Theo Colborn, et. al. *Our Stolen Future: A Medical Detective Story*, (Penguin Books, 1997)